A Handbook for Surgical Approaches to
Maxillofacial Trauma

A Handbook for Surgical Approaches to **Maxillofacial Trauma**

Rajesh Yadav MS DORL FCPS
Assistant Professor
Department of Otolaryngology, Head & Neck Surgery
Bhagwati Hospital
Mumbai, Maharashtra, India

Co-authors

Rashu Mittal MS (ENT)
Senior Resident
Department of Otolaryngology, Head & Neck Surgery
Shatabdi Hospital
Mumbai, Maharashtra, India

Prakash V Dhond MS (ENT)
Senior Consultant
Ex-Honorary Surgeon
Department of Otolaryngology, Head & Neck Surgery
Bhagwati Hospita
Mumbai, Maharashtra, India

Forewords

KP Morwani
Parag Kerkar

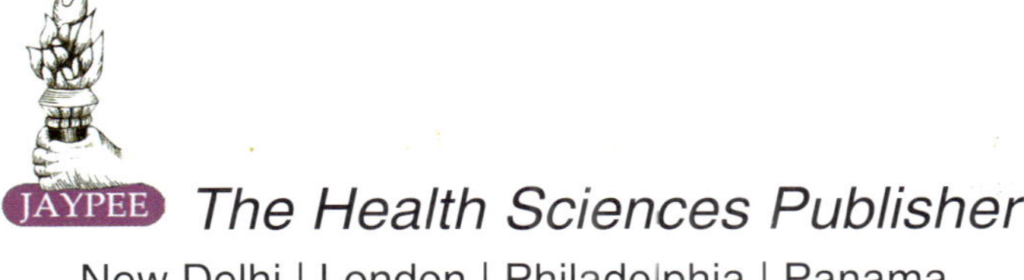

The Health Sciences Publisher
New Delhi | London | Philadelphia | Panama

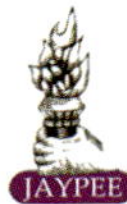

Jaypee Brothers Medical Publishers (P) Ltd

Headquarters
Jaypee Brothers Medical Publishers (P) Ltd
4838/24, Ansari Road, Daryaganj
New Delhi 110 002, India
Phone: +91-11-43574357
Fax: +91-11-43574314
Email: jaypee@jaypeebrothers.com

Overseas Offices

J.P. Medical Ltd
83, Victoria Street, London
SW1H 0HW (UK)
Phone: +44 20 3170 8910
Fax: +44 (0)20 3008 6180
Email: info@jpmedpub.com

Jaypee Medical Inc
325 Chestnut Street
Suite 412, Philadelphia, PA 19106, USA
Phone: +1 267-519-9789
Email: support@jpmedus.com

Jaypee Brothers Medical Publishers (P) Ltd
Bhotahity, Kathmandu, Nepal
Phone: +977-9741283608
Email: kathmandu@jaypeebrothers.com

Jaypee-Highlights Medical Publishers Inc
City of Knowledge, Bld. 237, Clayton
Panama City, Panama
Phone: +1 507-301-0496
Fax: +1 507-301-0499
Email: cservice@jphmedical.com

Jaypee Brothers Medical Publishers (P) Ltd
17/1-B, Babar Road, Block-B, Shaymali
Mohammadpur, Dhaka-1207
Bangladesh
Mobile: +08801912003485
Email: jaypeedhaka@gmail.com

Website: www.jaypeebrothers.com
Website: www.jaypeedigital.com

Inquiries for bulk sales may be solicited at: jaypee@jaypeebrothers.com

A Handbook for Surgical Approaches to Maxillofacial Trauma

First Edition: **2016**

ISBN 978-93-85891-55-7

Printed at: Sanat Printers

Dedicated to

My Late grandfather Shitla Prasad Yadav
&
My beloved brother, Late Dinesh Yadav
Who are still there with me and in me
Their sweet memory always keeps them alive
I miss them at every step of my life

—Rajesh Yadav

Foreword

Maxillofacial trauma was managed mainly by maxillofacial surgeon and plastic surgeon in past. Since last few decades, many ENT surgeons in the Western world have also specialized in this specialty.

Dr Rajesh Yadav was fortunate to work in Sir JJ Group of Hospital, Mumbai, under Dr Mohan Jagade, who is one of the few ENT surgeons who has done masters in plastic surgery; and, subsequently, Dr Rajesh Yadav was attached to peripheral Municipal General Hospital, Mumbai, where no plastic or maxillofacial surgeon was attached. He started his journey in this field by managing simple cases of fractured mandible; and with the help of plastic and maxillofacial colleagues, he has diversified in managing various pan-facial traumas. It has been gradual learning curve for him.

Three years back, he had published his first monogram on fracture mandible and now he is coming with his new manuscript *A Handbook for Surgical Approaches to Maxillofacial Trauma.*

He has taken extensive care to write this handbook in very simple language and explained each and every procedure in detail with simple diagrams.

I consider him as pioneer ENT surgeon in this field as very few ENT surgeons have diversified to this superspecialty. In fact, he has organized the first maxillofacial trauma hands-on course with live dissection with the help of Dr Mohan Jagade in March 2015 in Sir JJ Group of Hospital, Mumbai.

This is a good handbook for the beginners and practitioners who want to indulge in this superspecialty.

I wish him all the success for popularizing this specialty.

KP Morwani MS (ENT)
Consultant ENT and Skull Base Surgeon
Nanawati Hospital and Hiranandani Hospital
Ex-Honorary Surgeon
Bhagwati Hospital
Mumbai, Maharashtra, India

Foreword

It is a matter of great pride and honor to write a foreword for this book. This book represents conclusion of years of contribution to the field of maxillofacial surgery. The book by far is the most concise and precise. Synopsis of the concept in doing even the most complicated maxillofacial surgeries. I must say it is a must-read for young aspiring surgeons as well as good brush-up for the veterans who want to catch-up on the newer concepts. This book is a very sincere effort by Dr Rajesh Yadav, a surgeon par excellence himself to unbiasedly portray a simplified yet effective way of managing cases in maxillofacial region.

I wish him all the very best for his present and future endeavors and I am sure, this book will be an asset and a great contribution to the field of maxillofacial surgery.

Parag Kerkar
MDS (Oromaxillofacial Surgery)
Honorary Surgeon
Department of Otolaryngology, Head & Neck Surgery
Bhagwati Hospital
Mumbai, Maharashtra, India

Preface

After the wide acceptance of our first book *Fracture Mandible* and the constant inquiries from our colleagues, we decided to put forward our little experience with other facial fractures.

As the ENT branch is expanding its horizon by going into surrounding areas like ophthalmic, skull-base and cosmetic surgeries, we thought of pulling our efforts in compiling the work that we are doing in facial fractures.

Although management of these fractures are routinely and with expertise done by plastic and maxillofacial surgeons, peripheral hospitals like Bhagwati Hospital, Mumbai, where we practice and which is our temple, do not have the luxury of expert service of these branches. The trauma work which comes to our hospital initially forced us in this area but gradually we started enjoying the same.

As admitted in our first book, we do not claim that this is the only way but if our experience helps the people working in smaller town with poor infrastructure and without expertise of other branches, we will be happy.

We present herewith whatever we have learnt from our friends in different branches including our specialty who are doing this work for many years, with the addition of our little experience while working in Bhagwati Hospital, Shatabdi Hospital, Rajawadi Hospital and our private setup.

This is an overview and not a complete guide or a road map for treating the patients. But if this can generate interest in our colleagues to work in this area, our efforts have received the reward.

As learning does not stop at any level, we are ready to accept all the suggestions and criticism by our friends to fill the lacunae in this book. We are grateful to our teachers, paramedical staff and most importantly our patients who have shown confidence in us. We thank our family members to spare us for putting the efforts for the book.

We especially thank Dr KP Morwani, our *Guru* who kindly consented to write the foreword and blessed us.

Last but not least, we thank Shri Jitendar P Vij (Group Chairman), Mr Ankit Vij (Group President) and Mr Tarun Duneja (Director-Publishing) of M/s Jaypee Brothers Medical Publishers (P) Ltd, New Delhi, India, with their team of experts who have put in a lot of efforts are to be appreciated without words.

We hope all readers will like our efforts as our first book and bless us.

Rajesh Yadav
Rashu Mittal
Prakash V Dhond

Acknowledgments

Before I begin, I would like to express my gratefulness to God for all that He has given us; just cannot ask for more.

I would like to say thanks to my family members (my parents and kids) for constantly showering their blessings and love on me, Dr Akancha for being so sweet always and for her contribution in making all the schematic pictures for this book and Dr Payal Mittal for her idea of cover page theme for this book.

I would also like to say thanks to administrators Dr Mahendra Wadiwala, Dr Krishnakant Pimple; my seniors Dr Prakash V Dhond, Dr Lalit Seth, Dr Parag Kerkar, and my friend Dr Shashikant Mhashal, for their constant guidance and support, and staff and colleagues of Bhagwati and Shatabdi Hospitals, and most important our patients, for bestowing their trust on me and allowing me to treat them.

I would like to thank Dr Deepak More, Dr Narendra Sharma, Dr Sangam Pal and Dr Aprajita, for being my buddies and being always there for me.

Last but not least, I would like to express my heartfelt gratitude to Dr Megha, for being the fillip and impetus (directly or implicitly) for this book.

Thank you so much.

Indebted!

—Rajesh Yadav

Contents

Surgical Atlas

CHAPTER

Principles for Surgical Approaches to Maxillofacial Trauma

The success of any trauma surgery depends upon many factors. One being the adequate access and exposure of the trauma site. Surgery and manipulations are automatically simplified if trauma part is well-exposed. For exposure of surgical site, placement of incision is very much important. Incision can be very well placed near the area of interest with retraction of vessels and nerves as done in orthopedic surgeries, and the trauma part is addressed thereafter. This gives a lot of leverage to orthopedic surgeons as little regard is paid to aesthetic part, allowing them more flexibility in location, direction and length of incision placement. But our being the area of facial skeleton where such direct incisions cannot be placed as facial aesthetics has to be taken care of.

The primary factor in placement of our incisions is not surgical convenience but facial aesthetics. Placing incision anywhere on the face can lead to conspicuous scar leading to cosmetic deformity. Thus, all of the facial incisions are placed in incospicuous area. Sometimes incision is placed at very distant area from the site of fracture. For example, coronal incision is taken for nose and zygomatic arch repair (Fig. 1). This is purely done in the interest of cosmesis.

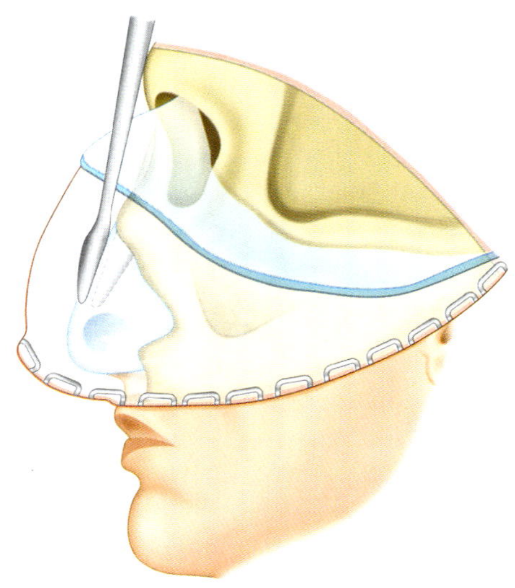

Fig. 1: Coronal approach used for reduction of nose and zygoma fracture

Another factor in the placement of our incision is presence of nerves and muscles of facial expression. Utmost care should be taken that the nerve supplying to the adjacent muscle is not traumatized if incision is placed in its path. This can lead to paralyzed face which not only gives cosmetic deformity but fuctional disabilities as well. For example, in preauricular incision which is used for the exposure of temporomandibular joint (TMJ), an oblique vertical incision is taken in temporalis fascia to prevent injury to frontal branch of facial nerve (Fig. 2).

Likewise, incision is placed 2 cm below the lower border of mandible to prevent injury to rama mandibularis (Figs 3A and B).

Third factor in facial incision placement is presence of many sensory nerves which exit from skull at multiple location. Thus, incision and approach used should be tailored to avoid injury to sensory nerves. For example:

- Dissection of supraorbital nerve from its foramen/notch in coronal approach (Fig. 4)
- Dissection of mental nerve in intraoral vestibular approach to symphysis and parasymphysis fractures (Fig. 5)
- Dissection of infraorbital nerve in maxillary vestibular approach (Fig. 6).

Other factors are:

- Age of the patient
- Existing unique anatomy
- Tendency of patient
- Expectation of patient.

Age

Age of the patient is important as possible presence of wrinkles in advancing age may serve as a guide and offer the surgeon oppurtunity to place the incision within or parallel to them.

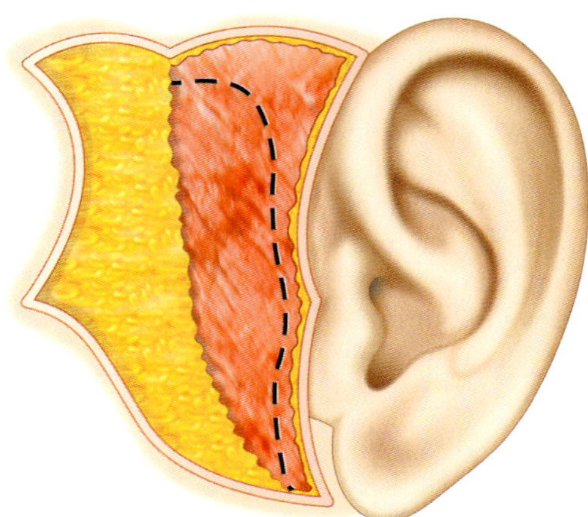

Fig. 2: Oblique vertical incision in temporalis fascia to prevent injury to frontal branch of facial nerve

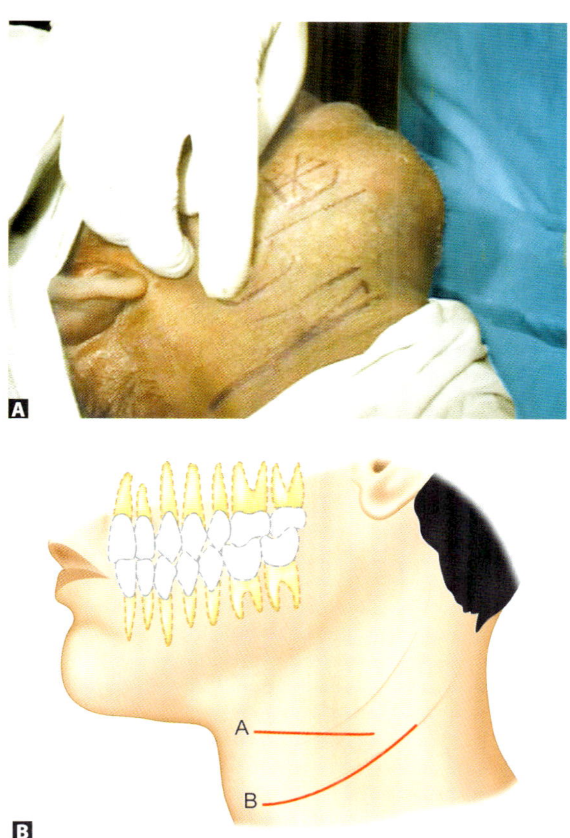

Figs 3A and B: Incision placed 2 cm below the body of mandible to prevent injury to marginal mandibular nerve

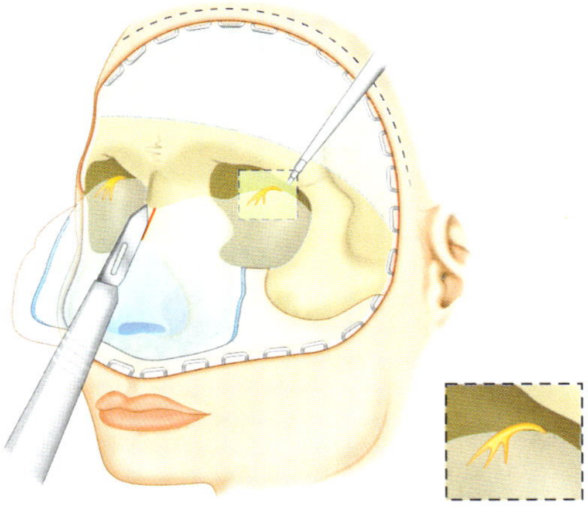

Fig. 4: Dissection of supraorbital nerve from its foramen in coronal approach

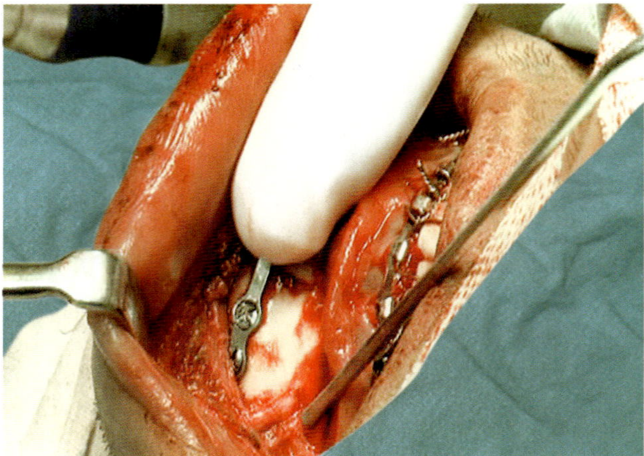

Fig. 5: Preservation of mental nerve in intraoral vestibular approach

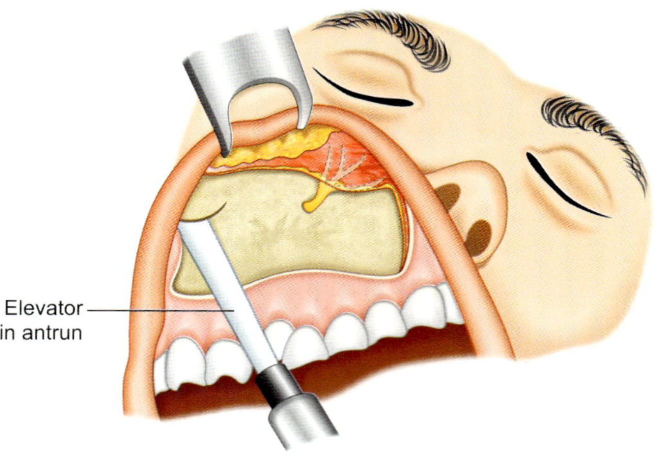

Fig. 6: Preservation of infraorbital nerve in maxillary vestibular approach

Existing Unique Anatomy

Unique anatomy of an individual can facilitate or hamper placement of incision. For example, pre-existing laceration can be used themselves or can be extended to provide surgical exposure to the underlying skeleton (Figs 7A and B).

Incision can be placed directly over an existing old scar. If it is ugly then the scar can be revised and same can be used for placement of the incision.

Position of the hair line determines the placement of incision. For example, incision used in coronal approach largely depends upon the position of hair line (Figs 8A and B).

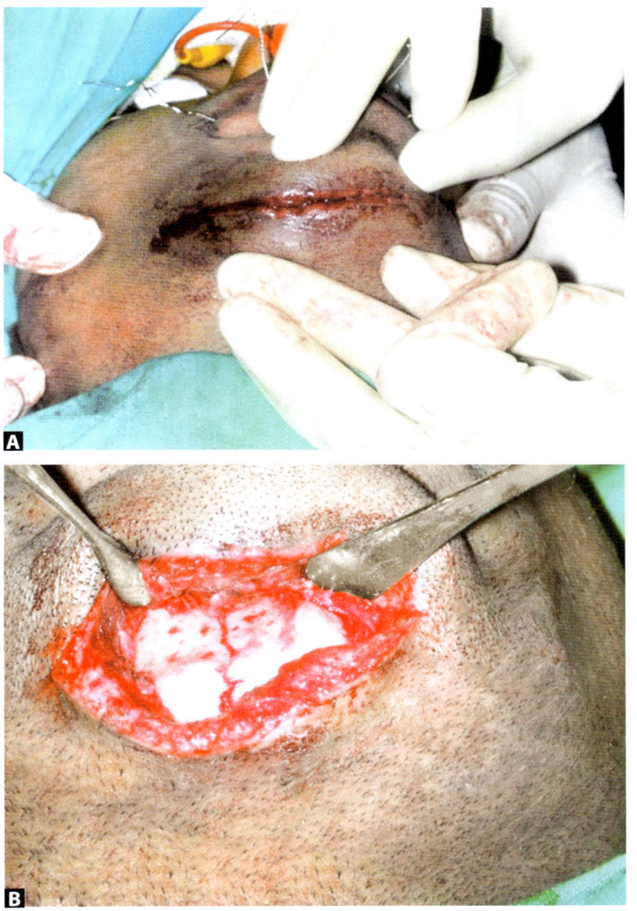

Figs 7A and B: Use of preexisting laceration to approach underlying fracture

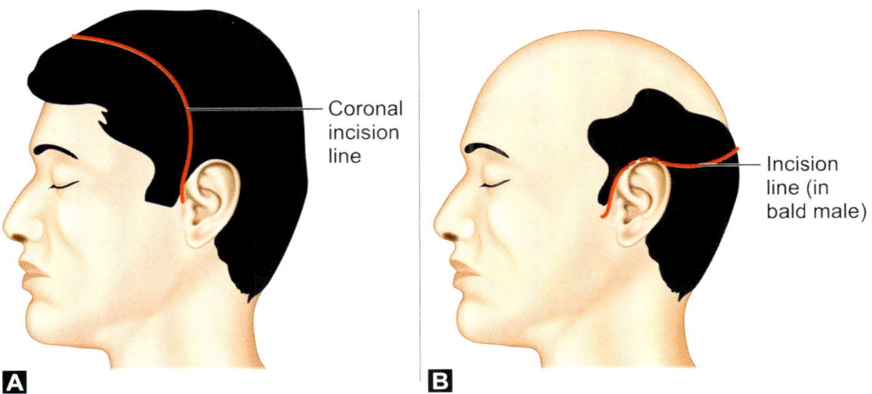

Figs 8A and B: Showing placement of incision according to hair line. Incision is placed few millimeters behind the hair line

Tendency of the Patient

Some patients have tendency for hypertrophic scar or keloid formation, hypo- or hyperpigmentation after trauma or incision. This should be considered prior to placement of the incision.

Expectations of the Patient

Wish and expectations of a patient determines the placement of the incision. For example, facelift incision is used for subcondylar fractures who wish to have an inconspicuous scar (Fig. 9).

PRINCIPLES OF INCISION PLACEMENT

Always try to use incision which is not visible or hidden in the hair line but compromise in exposure should not be done. If incision is placed over exposed surface, some basic principles are to be followed so that the scar becomes less visible. These principles are:

Avoid Injury to Important Neurovascular Structure

The important neurovascular structures encountered during the dissection should be dealt carefully. Utmost care must be taken during dissection around these neurovascular bundles and least pressure should be exerted while retracting them.

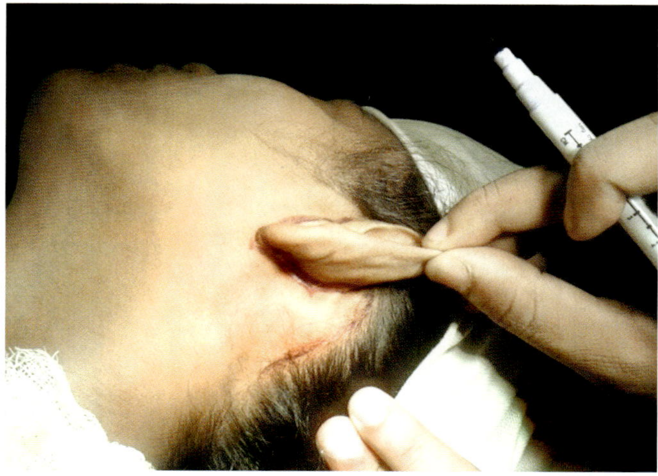

Fig. 9: Facelift incision for subcondylar fracture

Use of Long and Adequate Incision as Necessary

Instead of placing a short incision and overstreching the soft tissue, it is always better to have a well-placed long incision which requires less retraction. A long incision heals as quickly as short ones so little extension of incision does not make any big difference.

Place Incision Perpendicular to the Surface of Non-hair Bearing Skin

The incision is always placed perpendicular to the skin surface as it permits wound margin to be reapproximated in accurate layer-to-layer fashion.

If the incision is placed oblique to the skin, such incision have chances of marginal necrosis and overlapping of edges during closure.

Incision in a hair bearing tissue should always be parallel to the direction of the hair so that only few follicles are sacrificed.

Incision Placed in the Line of Mimimum Tension

There are lines of minimum tension also known as relaxed skin tension line which are seen over aged faces. Incision along these creases causes scar which is imperceptible (Fig. 10).

If the incision cannot be placed in the line of minimum tension then this can be made inconspicuous by placing them inside the orifice such as mouth, nose or eyelid or within hair bearing area.

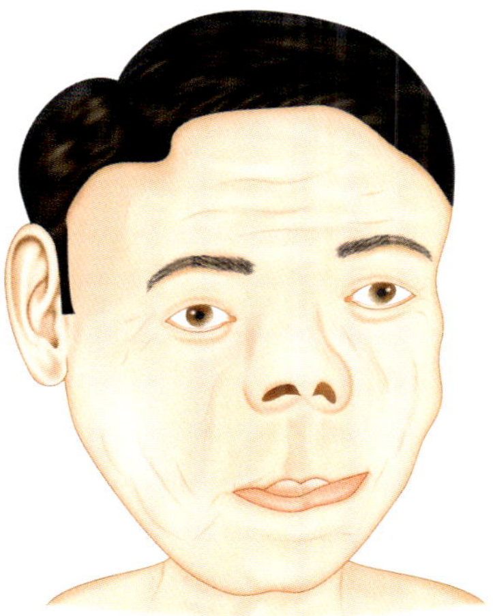

Fig. 10: Lines of minimum tension

NEWER TECHNIQUES

With the advent of endoscopes and expertise of ENT surgeons over endoscopes, endoscopic approaches are very well used for management of various skeletal fractures.

For example, management of depressed frontal bone fracture may not require coronal approach or brow incision. This can be very well-managed by endoscopic approach.

Nowadays management of orbital floor fracture, medial wall orbital fracture, etc. has been drastically changed shifting from conventional open procedures to more conservative endonasal endoscopic approaches.

Approaches to Airways

Most of the maxillofacial trauma cases require nasal intubation. The reason behind the preference for nasal intubation is:
- The tube does not come in a way of mouth opening and closing
- Occlusion can be checked frequently.

But at times nasal intubation may be difficult and can be contraindicated. For example, in cases of:
- Nasal bone fracture
- Skull base injury.

Other options available in cases where nasal intubation cannot be done are:
1. Tracheostomy
2. Submental intubation
3. Retromolar intubation

TRACHEOSTOMY (FIG. 1)

Advantages

- All ENT surgeons are well-versed with tracheostomy
- It gives safe and secure airway
- Method of choice when long-term life support system is required (mechanical ventilation).

Disadvantages

- Separate incision is required
- Invasive technique
- Require good postopertive care
- Chances of injury to important neck structures

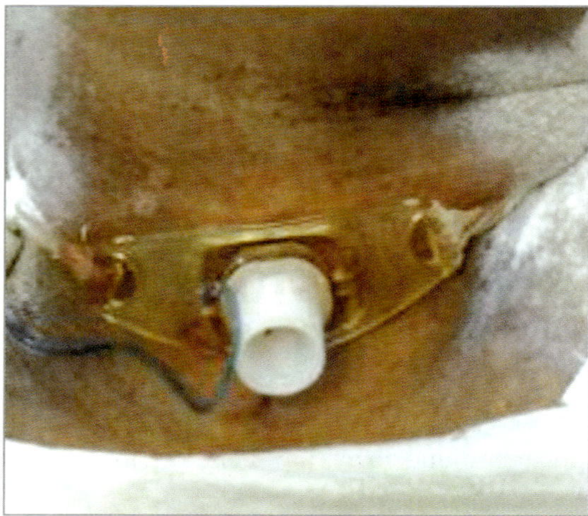

Fig. 1: Tracheostomy tube in-situ

- Hemorrhage
- Subglottic stenosis
- Difficulty in speech and swallowing.

SUBMENTAL INTUBATION

It is an alternative method for tracheal intubation.

Indications

- Cases of skull base trauma
- Nasal bone fracture along with panfacial trauma
- Cases in which tracheostomy has to be avoided.

Advantages

- Combined advantage of nasotracheal and orotracheal intubation
- Frequent dental occlusion can be checked during this intubation
- Frontonasal areas can be assessed properly
- Avoid the risk of iatrogenic meningitis and trauma to anterior skull base.

Limitations

- Cannot be used for patients with neurological deficits
- Cannot be used for thoracic trauma patients
- Patients requiring long-standing mechanical ventilation
- Patient requiring multiple operations.

Disadvantages

- External scar is given as it is an extraoral procedure
- Special armoured tube is required for intubation
- Special expertise is required
- Chances of dislodgement of tube is higher, hence anesthetist needs to be more vigilant.

Procedure

- Patient is intubated orally with armoured tracheal tube
- Prior to this the universal connector must be removed or cut off and replaced with a removable connector to allow easy detachment
- Using an aseptic technique, lower part of neck and face is painted with an appropriate antiseptic solution
- A 1.5 cm skin crease incision is made in the submental region (Fig. 2A), just medial to the lower border of the mandible, approximately one-third of the way from the symphysis to the angle of the mandible
- Incision is usually taken on the same side of the fracture
- Mouth opening is maintained using a gag or dental prop and the tongue is retracted, exposing the floor of the mouth
- A medium-sized curved artery forceps is then introduced into the submental incision (Fig. 2B) and blunt dissection is carried out towards the floor of the mouth, staying as close as possible to the inner (lingual) aspect of the mandible to avoid damaging the sublingual gland, submandibular duct and lingual nerve.

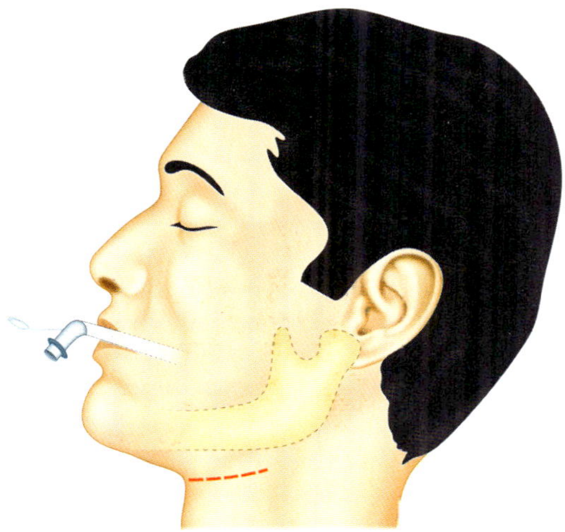

Fig. 2A: Submental incision

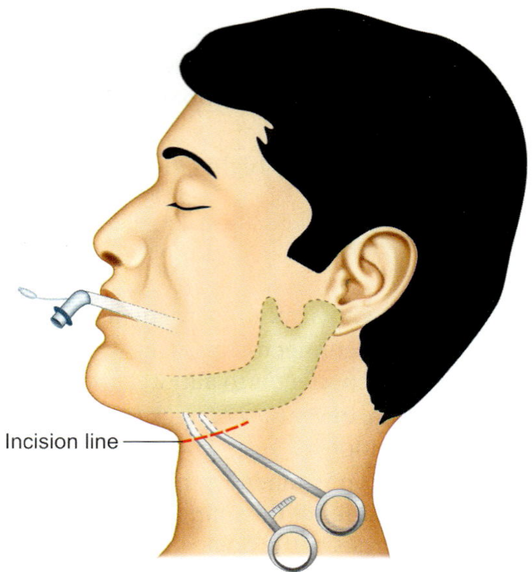

Fig. 2B: Dissection continued to approach floor of mouth

The tissue encountered are:

- Skin
- Subcutaneous fat
- Platysma
- Investing layer of deep cervical fascia
- Mylohyoid muscle
- Mucosa of floor of mouth.

The oral mucosa is tented with a hemostat from submental wound. Now an incision is taken along this tented mucosa at the attached margin of gingiva. At this stage, connector of the armored tube is detached (Fig. 2C).

With the help of a mosquito, the oral tube is delivered through submental wound (Fig. 2D).

The position of the tracheal tube is checked using capnography and chest auscultation and a careful note is made of the marking on the tube at the skin exit site as there is always a chance of accidental extubation.

The tube is then secured to the skin of the submental region with adhesive tape or sutured with black silk.

Complications

- Chances of infection
- Chances of orocutaneous fistula

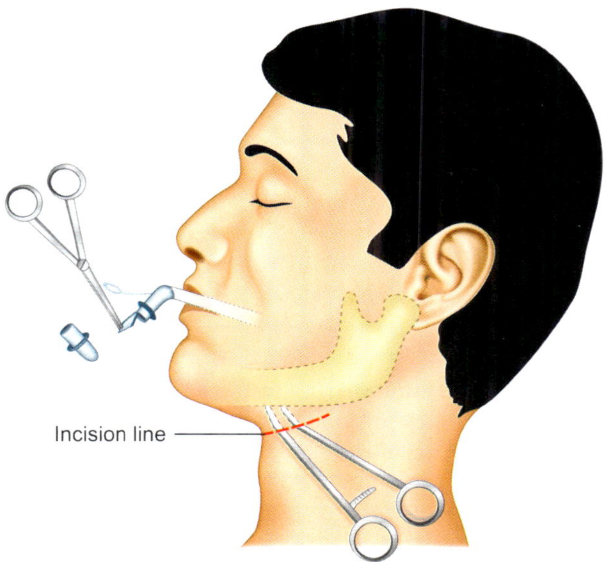

Fig. 2C: Detachment of connector from armored tube

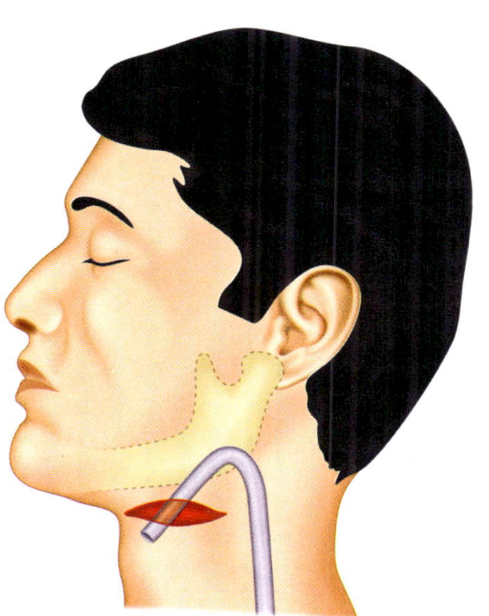

Fig. 2D: Delivery of tube through submental wound

- Chances of scar formation
- Injury to submental vessels (branches of facial vessels) can lead to hemorrhage
- Chances of accidental extubation
- Chances of duct injury
- Chances of wound dehiscence
- Transient lingual nerve paresthesia
- Mucocele formation.

RETROMOLAR INTUBATION

It is another noninvasive technique for securing the airways in patients with panfacial trauma. It avoids the complications of tracheostomy and submental intubation.

Advantages

- Better technique over tracheostomy and submental intubation
- Lesser rate of complication
- Noninvasive
- Less time consumption.

Limitations and Disadvantages

- Requires a special fiberoptic tube
- Not a dependable technique as retromolar space may not be adequate in all the patients
- Tracheal tube may interfere with surgical manipulation
- Chances of tube getting deformed due to tight fixation.

Anatomical Consideration

- *Retromolar space (Fig. 3A):* Located between distal aspect of last mandibular molar and anterior edge of ascending ramus
- *Superior:* Maxillary tuberosity and area behind the tuberosity (retrotuberosity area)
- *Inferiorly:* Retromolar trigone area
- *Anteriorly:* 3rd molar
- *Posteriorly:* Anterior border of ascending ramus
- *Medially:* Lateral surface of tuberosity and last erupted molar
- *Laterally:* Medial surface of ascending ramus and buccal vestibule.

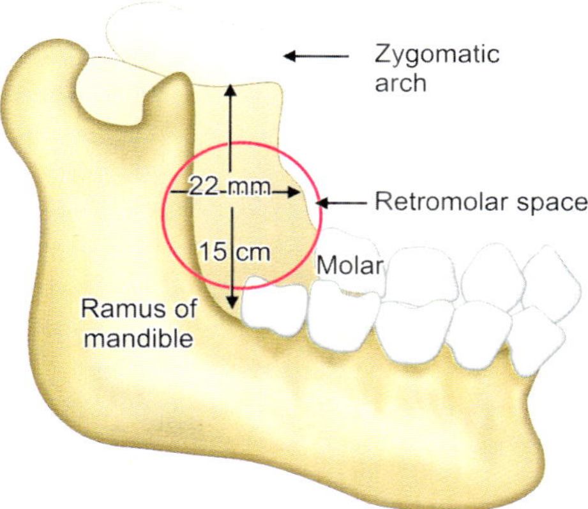

Fig. 3A: Boundaries of retromolar space

This retromolar space may be insufficient in many patients. The space is determined by:

- Eruption status of molar teeth
- Impaction of 3rd molar.

So before considering retromolar intubation one needs to check the adequacy of space.

Checking Adequacy of Space

A gloved index finger is placed in the retromolar space and patient is asked to close the mouth slowly. If there is no compression over the finger that suggest enough retromolar space. Though easy but this method cannot be relied upon. This test cannot be performed in uncoopertive patients and childern.

- An orthopentogram may be useful to assess the retromolar space.

Technique

Orotracheal intubation is done initially with a flexometallic tracheal tube using standard general anesthesia technique.

The orotracheal tube is grasped with gloved fingers and is placed into the retromolar space (Fig. 3B). The retromolar tracheal tube allows adequate dental occlusion (Fig. 3C), thus rendering intraoperative intermaxillary fixation feasible.

At the end of surgical procedure, intermaxillary fixation (IMF) is opened resulting in adequate mouth opening.

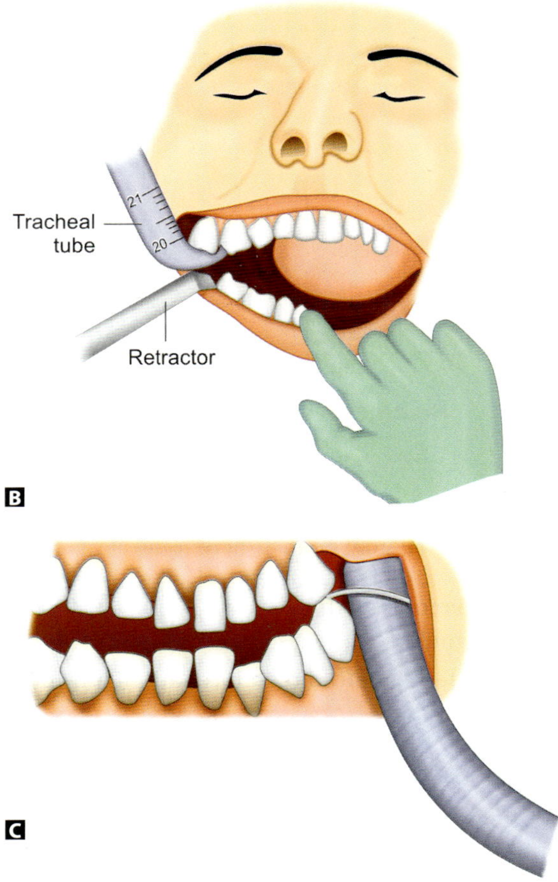

Figs 3B and 3C: Introduction of tube through retromolar space and checking for dental occlusion

The retromolar tracheal tube is converted back to orotracheal tube. Subsequently, trachea is extubated by the standard method.

CHAPTER

Occlusion and Buttress

One of the basic principles of any oral-maxillofacial surgery is to restore a normal occlusion or preexisting occlusion.

WHAT IS OCCLUSION?

Occlusion is a mixture of two words; "clusion" means "closing" and the prefix "oc" means "up", and thus it means "closing up".

Basically, occlusion is referred to a relationship of maxillary and mandibular tooth when they are in functional contact during the activities of mandible.

Since, occlusal relationship of tooth is an important determinant, hence we need to know the basics of dental anatomy.

The dental arch is divided into two arches, i.e. upper and lower dental arches (maxillary and mandibular arch). Each arch is then further subdivided into right and left quadrant by an arbitrary vertical line. The vertical line passes through maxillary and mandibular central incisiors. Thus, dental arch is divided into four quadrants:

1. 1st right upper (maxillary arch)
2. 2nd left upper (maxillary arch)
3. 3rd left lower (mandibular arch)
4. 4th right lower (mandibular arch).

Types of Teeth

Teeth are divided into anterior and posterior teeth.

- Anterior teeth—their function is cutting and tearing of food
- Posterior teeth—they help in grinding and chewing of food.

Identification of Teeth

To understand occlusion, it is very much important for us to identify individual tooth. Basically, we have four types of tooth:

1. Incisor
2. Canine
3. Premolar
4. Molar

Incisors and canines are considered as anterior teeth whereas premolars and molars are included into posterior teeth.

1. *Incisors:* There are four incisors in each arch, i.e. central and lateral incisors. They look like a chisel and are used for cutting or incising the food (Fig. 1).

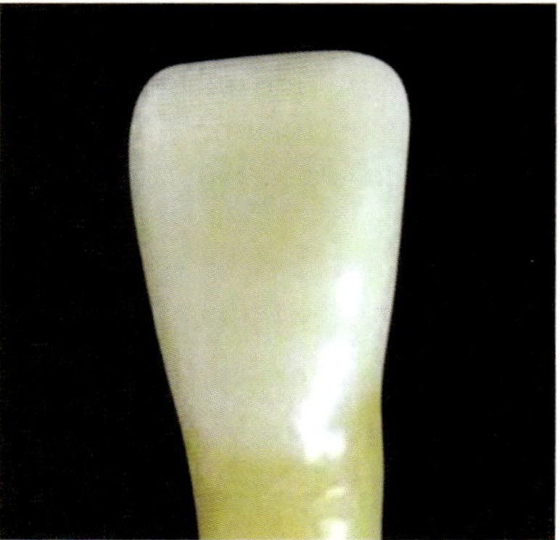

Fig. 1: Incisor

2. *Canine:* There are two canines in each arch. They are wedge-shaped and help in cutting and tearing the food (Fig. 2).

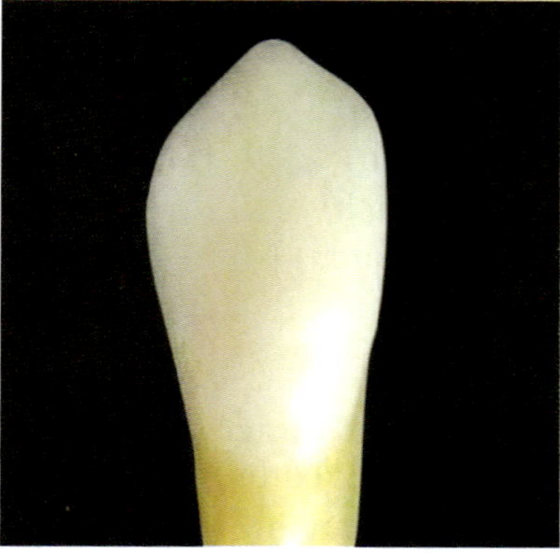

Fig. 2: Canine

3. *Premolars:* There are four premolars in each arch (in adults). They have got atleast two cusps (projections) and helps in tearing and grinding of food (Fig. 3).

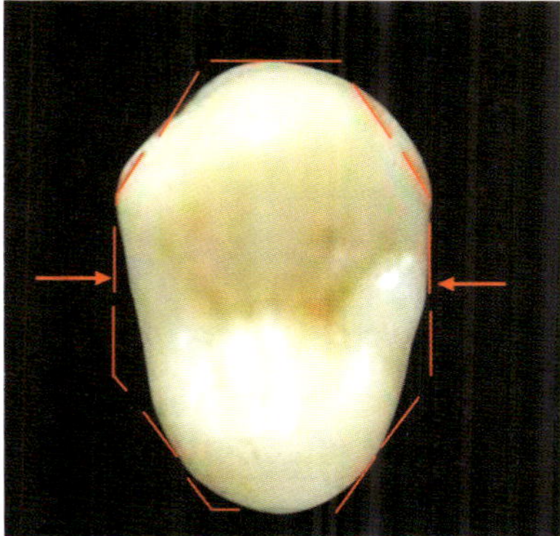

Fig. 3: Premolar

4. *Molars:* There are six molars in each arch (in adults). They have got multiple cusps (projections) and helps mainly in grinding of food (Fig. 4).

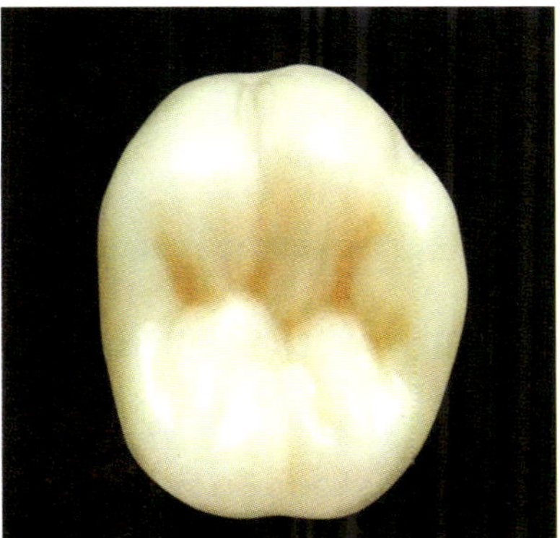

Fig. 4: Molar

Tooth Identification System

There are various tooth numbering systems for designation of each tooth:

1. Palmer notation system
2. Universal system
3. International FDI system (two digit system)

In India, the most commonly used system is Federation Dentaire International (FDI) system. In FDI system, teeth are designated by two-digit.

a. The **first digit** of the code is located at the left side of the number and indicates the **quadrant** (Fig. 5).

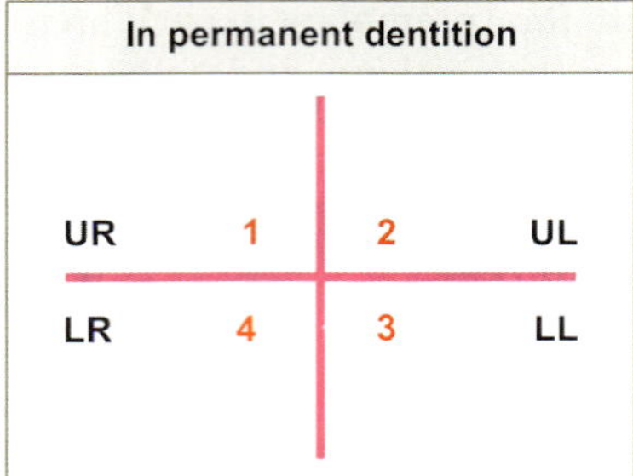

Fig. 5: FDI notation system. numbers indicating the respective quadrant (UR, upper right; UL, upper left; LL, left lower; LR, left right)

b. The **second digit** is located at the right side of the number and indicates the number of the tooth in the **quadrant** (Fig. 6).

In permanent dentition															
18	17	16	15	14	13	12	11	21	22	23	24	25	25	26	27	28
48	47	46	45	44	43	42	41	31	32	33	34	35	35	36	37	38

Fig. 6: FDI notation system. Numbers on right indicate the respective tooth in each quadrant

The two digits should be pronounced separately.

Surfaces of Teeth

Surfaces of teeth are identified by their relationship to surrounding orofacial structures.

Each Tooth has Five Surfaces

1. *Facial:* Further subdivided into labial and buccal (Figs 7 and 8).
   - surface facing towards the lips is labial (for incisors and canines) and those facing towards buccal cavity are buccal (for premolars and molars)

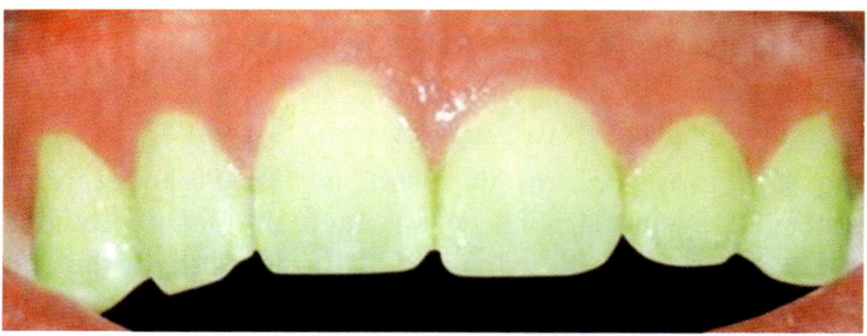

Fig. 7: Labial surface

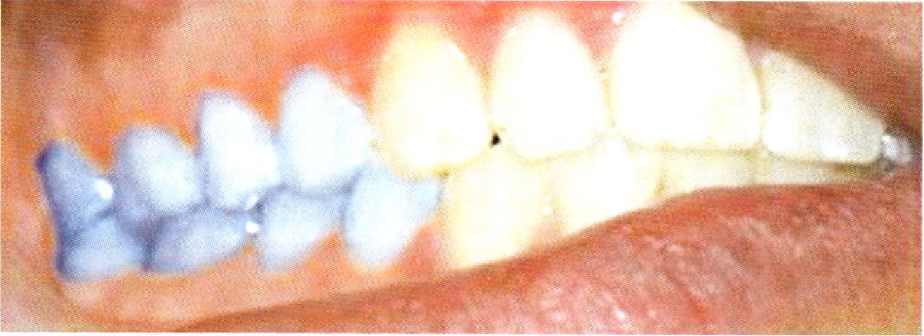

Fig. 8: Buccal surface

2. *Lingual/Palatal:* Surface facing toward the tongue is lingual surface (mandibular teeth) and those facing towards the palate are known as palatal (maxillary teeth) (Figs 9A and B).

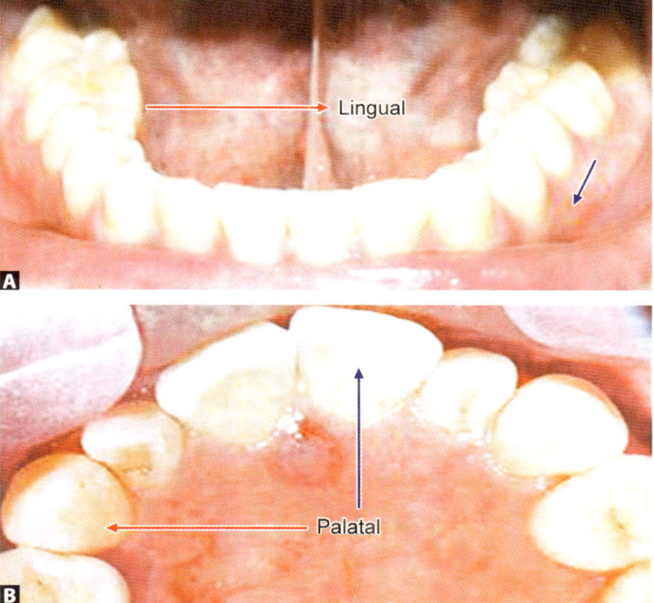

Figs 9A and B: (A) Lingual surface; (B) Palatal surface

3. *Mesial:* Surface facing toward the midline is mesial surface (Fig. 10).

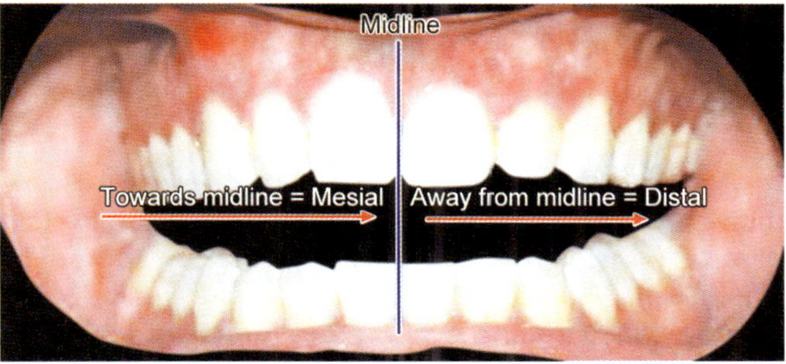

Fig. 10: Mesial and distal surfaces

4. *Distal:* Surface facing away from midline is distal surface (Fig. 11).
5. *Occlusal/Incisal:* Surface involved in biting or making occlusion is occlusal surface.
   - **Incisal** is used for anterior teeth, whereas occlusal are used for posterior teeth.

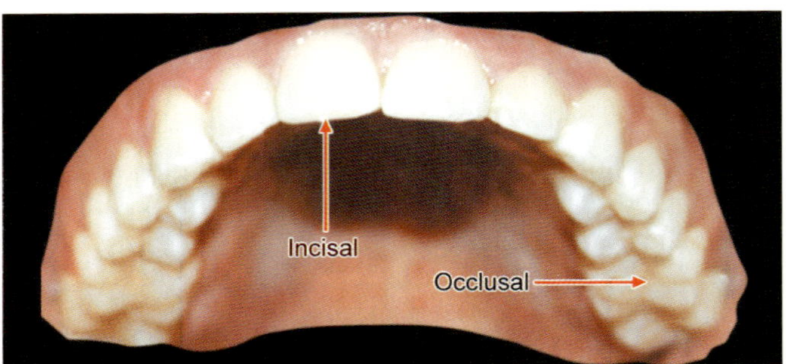

Fig. 11: Incisal and occlusal surfaces

NORMAL OCCLUSION

The mesiobuccal cusp of the maxillary first molar is aligned with the mesiobuccal groove of the mandibular first molar. There is slight overriding of maxillary incisors over mandibular incisors.

Malocclusion

Malocclusion is classified into three classes:

- *Class I:* A class I (neutral) occlusion is one in which the mesial buccal cusp of the upper first molar occludes with the mesial buccal groove of the mandibular first molar, means a normal molar relationship exists but there is crowding, misalignment of the teeth, cross bites, etc. (Fig. 12).

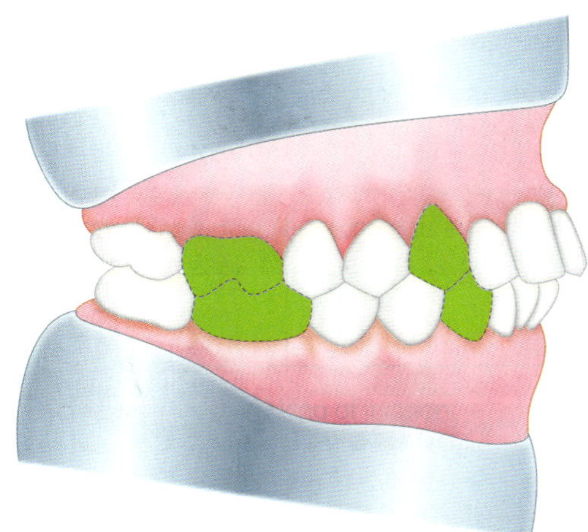

Fig. 12: Class I malocclusion

- *Class II:* A malocclusion where the molar relationship shows the buccal groove of the mandibular first molar distally positioned when in occlusion with the distobuccal cusp of the maxillary first molar (Fig. 13). This means mesiobuccal cusp of upper molar lies anterior to the mesiobuccal groove of the lower molar.

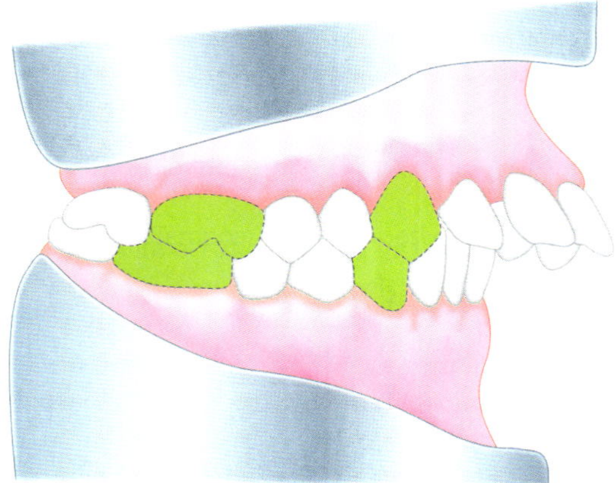

Fig. 13: Class II malocclusion

- *Class III:* A malocclusion where the molar relationship shows the mesiobuccal cusp of maxillary first molar occludes in the interdental space between the mandibular first and second molar means mesiobuccal cusp of upper molar comes posterior to the mesiobuccal groove of the lower molar when the teeth are in occlusion (Fig. 14).

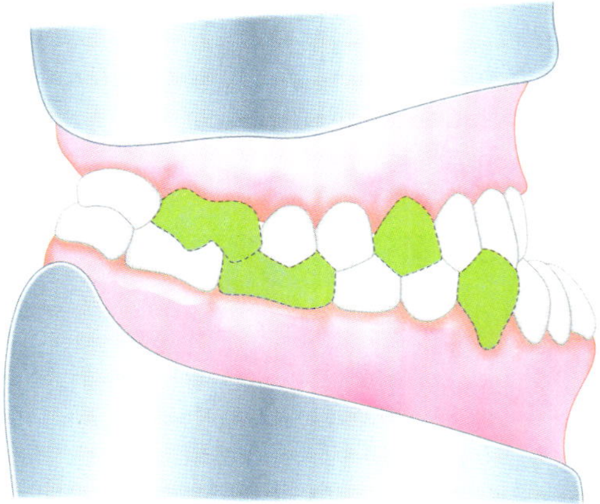

Fig. 14: Class III malocclusion

Identification of Preexisting Occlusion

The first step in identifying abnormal occlusal patterns is to count the teeth and identifying those that are missing and those that are present. Missing teeth in the partially dentulous patients can produce changes in dental relationship.

***Note:** A patient with class III occlusion before injury would be impossible to treat by attempting to force teeth into a neutral occlusion.

Guide to Proper Occlusion

Generally, molar relationship is used to achieve normal occlusion, but cases in which molars are missing we can use central incisors and canine teeth as the guiding tooth.

WEAR FACETS

- The preexisting occlusion can often easily be recognized by the wear facet
- Wear facets are the worn surface caused by repeated contact of maxillary and mandibular tooth
  - **Class I** often shows more wear surfaces on the outer (labial) edges of the mandibular anterior and on the under (lingual) surfaces of the maxillary anterior teeth
  - **Class II** usually has no wear facets on the incisor edges of the lower anterior teeth
  - **Class III** wear facet on the outer anterior edge of the maxillary teeth.

Malocclusions

Open Bite

An open bite is when there is no vertical overlap between maxillary and mandibular teeth (Fig. 15).

a. Anterior open bite:

- Conditions in which anterior open bite is encountered:
  - Bilateral condylar fracture (Fig. 16)
  - Bilateral angle fracture
  - Le Fort fracture (Fig. 17)

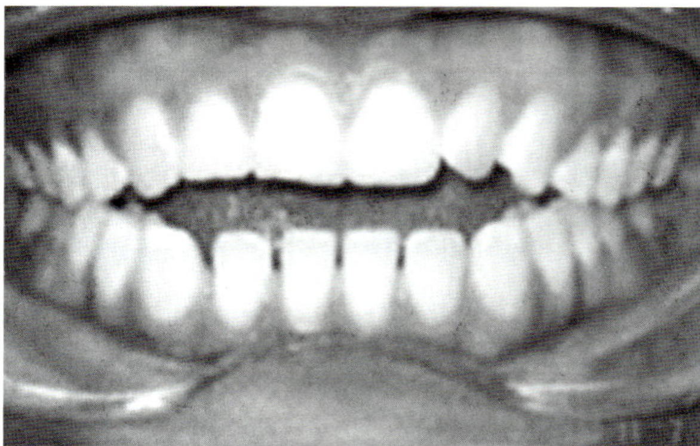

Fig. 15: Anterior open bite

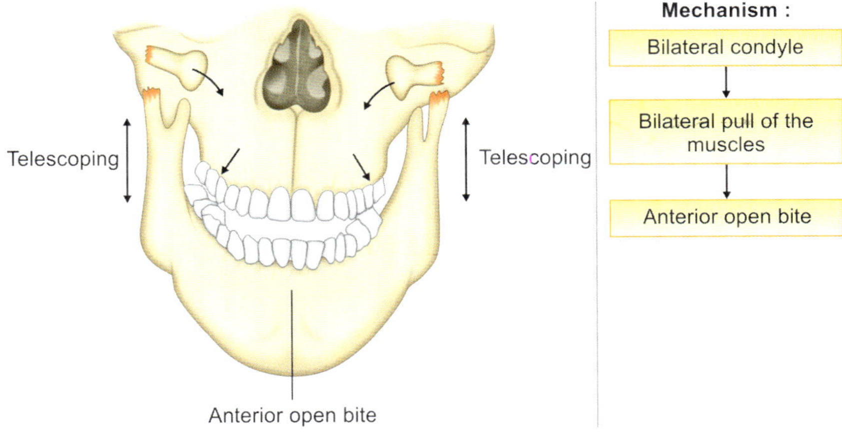

Fig. 16: Bilateral condylar fracture (below the attachment of lateral pterygoid)

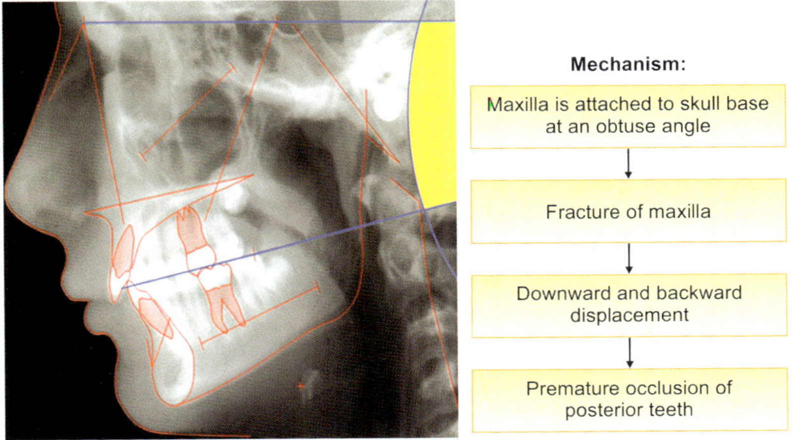

Fig. 17: Le Fort fracture

b. Posterior open bite (Fig. 18):

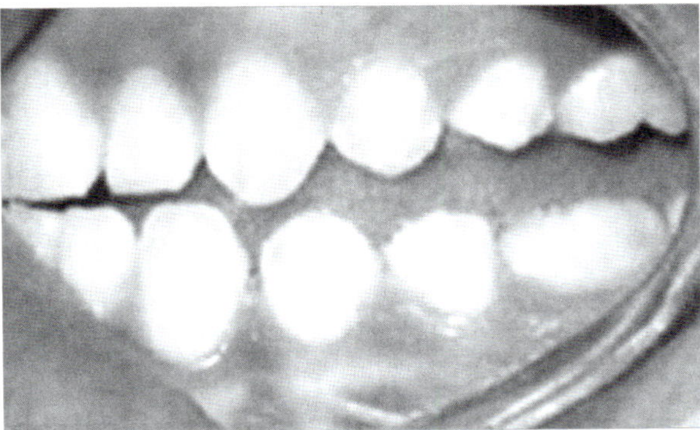

Fig. 18: Posterior open bite

- Condition in which posterior open bite are encountered:
  - Contralateral condylar fracture (Figs 19 and 20)
  - Ipsilateral angle fracture

A. Mechanism of condylar fracture (below the attachment of lateral pterygoid)

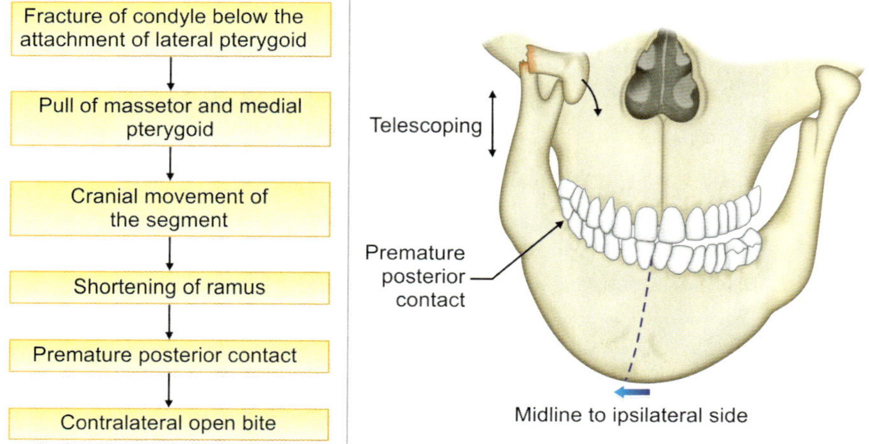

Fig. 19: Unilateral condylar fracture

B. Mechanism of condylar fracture (above the attachment of lateral pterygoid)

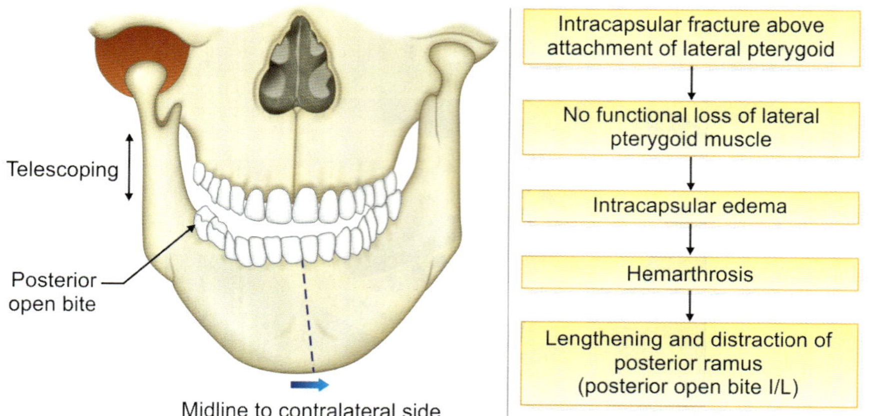

Fig. 20: Effusion hemarthrosis

Cross Bite

It is a form of malocclusion where a tooth (or teeth) has a more buccal or lingual position (i.e. the tooth is either closer to the cheek or to the tongue) than its corresponding antagonist tooth in the upper or lower dental arch.

a. Anterior cross-bite (Fig. 21):

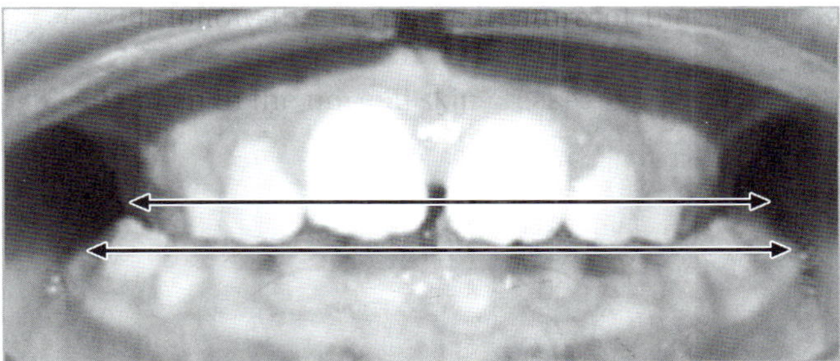

Fig. 21: Anterior cross-bite

b. Posterior cross-bite (Fig. 22):

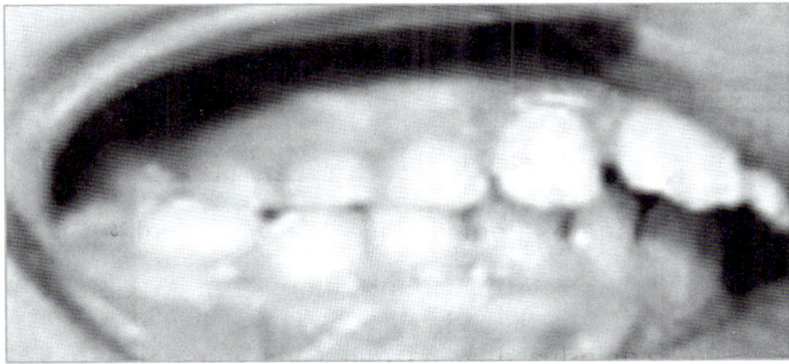

Fig. 22: Posterior cross-bite

Buttresses

A buttress is an architectural structure built against or projecting from a wall which serves to support or reinforce the wall.

The facial skeleton receives support and stability from a series of transverse and vertical facial buttresses. Facial buttresses represent areas of thick bone that support the surrounding thinner facial bones, sustain masticatory forces, and protect vital structures. Restoration of facial width, height, and projection is achieved by reducing and reconstructing the facial buttresses.

Buttresses of the face are generally divided into vertical and horizontal planes.

Vertical Buttresses

The vertical buttresses include:

a. Nasomaxillary buttress
b. Zygomaticomaxillary buttress
c. Pterygomaxillary buttress

a. *Nasomaxillary buttress:* This includes the maxillary process of the frontal bone and the frontal process of the maxilla, extending lateral to the piriform rim (Fig. 23).

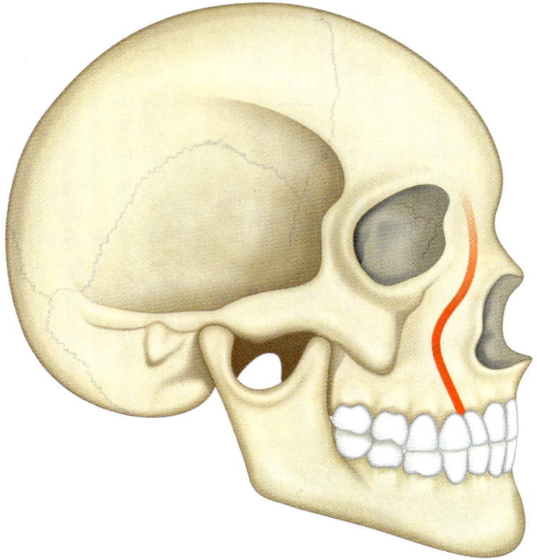

Fig. 23: Red mark showing nasomaxillary buttress

b. *Zygomaticomaxillary buttress:* This is composed of the zygomatic process of the frontal bone, lateral orbital rim, lateral zygomatic body, and zygomatic process of the maxilla (Fig. 24).

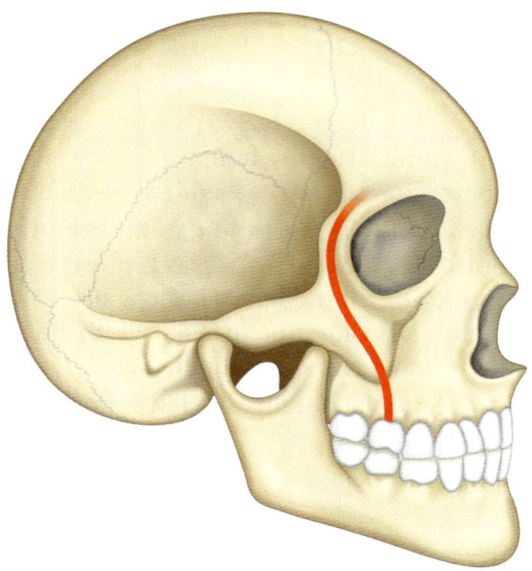

Fig. 24: Red mark showing zygomaticomaxillary buttress

c. *Pterygomaxillary buttress:* This includes the pterygoid plates of the sphenoid and maxillary tuberosities (Fig. 25).

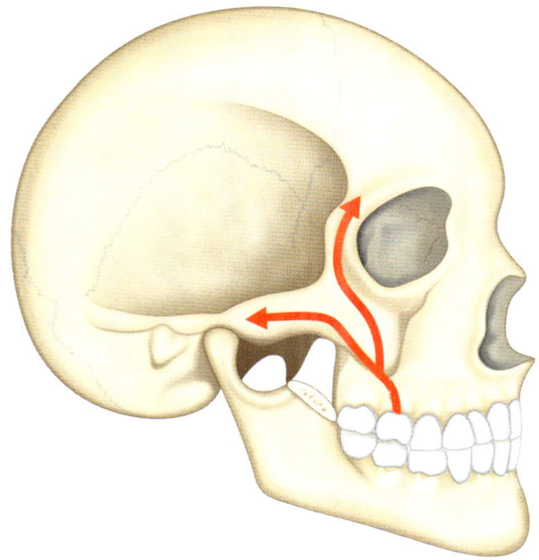

Fig. 25: Arrow mark depecting pterygcmaxillary buttress

Usually, the nasomaxillary and zygomaticomaxillary buttresses are reconstructed, but the pterygomaxillary buttress is not because of inaccessibility.

The condyle and posterior mandibular ramus make up yet another buttress establishing posterior facial height.

Horizontal Buttresses

The horizontal buttresses are also described as *anterior-posterior buttresses* (Fig. 26).

These include:

a. Frontal buttress
b. Zygomatic buttress
c. Maxillary buttress
d. Mandibular buttress.
    - The frontal buttress is composed of the supraorbital rims and the glabellar region
    - The zygomatic buttress consists of the zygomatic arch, zygomatic body, and infraorbital rim
    - The maxillary and mandibular buttresses are composed of the basal bone of the maxilla and mandiblar arches.

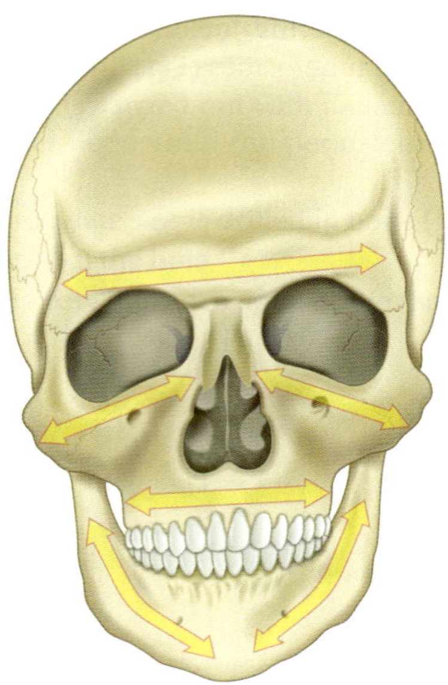

Fig. 26: Showing all the horizontal buttresses with yellow markings

Together, they give the facial skeleton its structural integrity. The bone is generally thicker over these described areas to neutralize the forces of mastication or impact. With the proper reduction of these buttresses, we are able to reconstruct the height, width, and projection of the face.

CHAPTER

Intermaxillary Fixation

There are various methods of immobilization. Most commonly in use are Erich arch bars.

ARCH BARS

Indications

- For a temporary fragment stabilization in cases of emergency
- As a method of closed reduction for simple fractures and condylar fractures
- It can be used for stabilization of alveolar fractures
- It can be used intraoperatively for maintaining occlusion
- It can be used for long-term fixation of comminuted, infected and edentulous fractures.

Advantages

- Easy technique
- Cost effective
- No special expertise required
- It can be done under local anesthesia
- It can be done in minor operation theater or bedside.

Disadvantages

- Chances of injury to soft tissue
- Risk of contamination of blood-borne infections.

Steps

- **Infiltration:** Two percent lignocaine with adrenaline is injected at upper and lower gingivobuccal sulcus
  - Mental nerve block given
  - Inferior alveolar nerve block given
- Appropriate size of arch bar is selected according to patient's dental arch (Figs 1A and B).

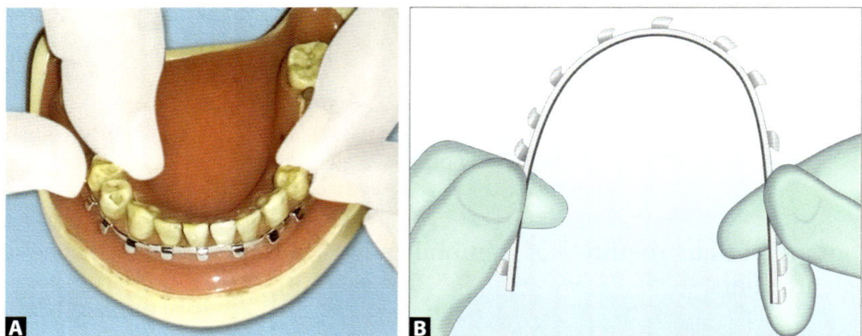

Figs 1A and B: Showing appropriate sized arch bar

- Arch bar is contoured on dental arch and cut accordingly. Extra length of arch bar needs to be cut (Figs 1C and D) and posterior edge of bar needs to be bent to prevent soft tissue injury.

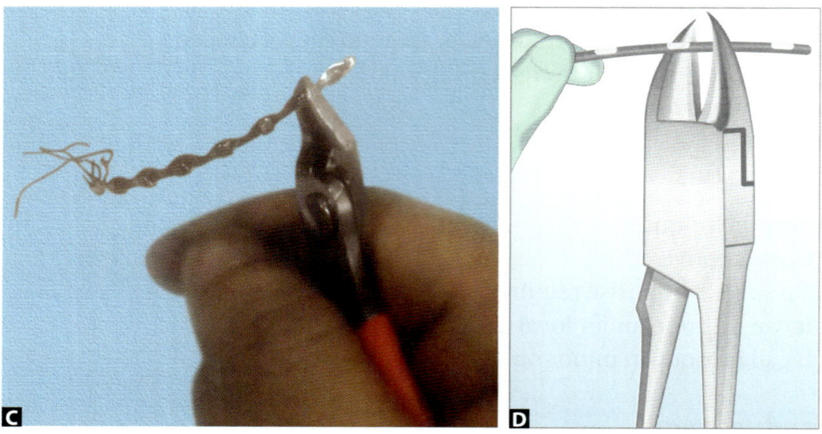

Figs 1C and D: Extra length of arch bar is cut

- Twenty six number wire is introduced through interdental space labially and is retrieved on lingual side (Fig. 2).

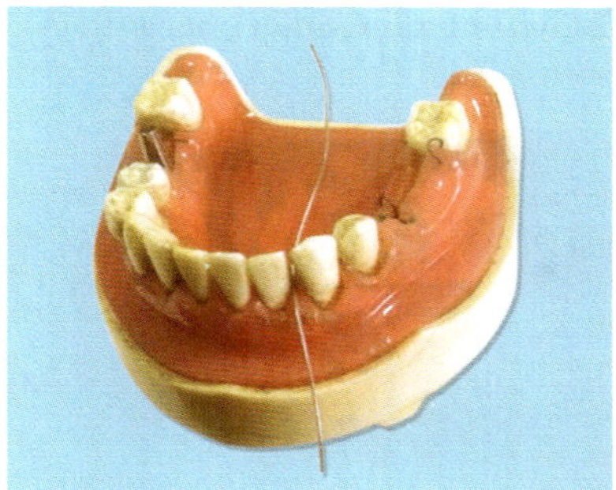

Fig. 2: Wire is passed through interdental space from labial to lingual side

- Wire is again introduced into adjacent interdental space from lingual side and retrieved again on labial side (Fig. 3).

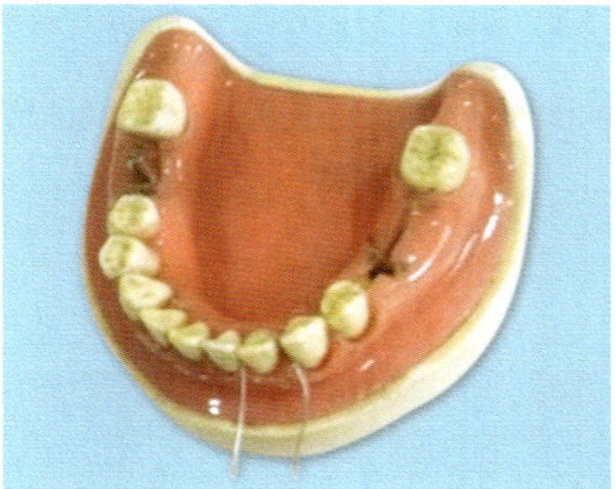

Fig. 3: Wire is retrieved from lingual to labial side through adjacent interdental space

- The wire is introduced in such a way that passes above and below the arch bar. Then with the help of twister the wire is twisted around the lug (Figs 4A and B).

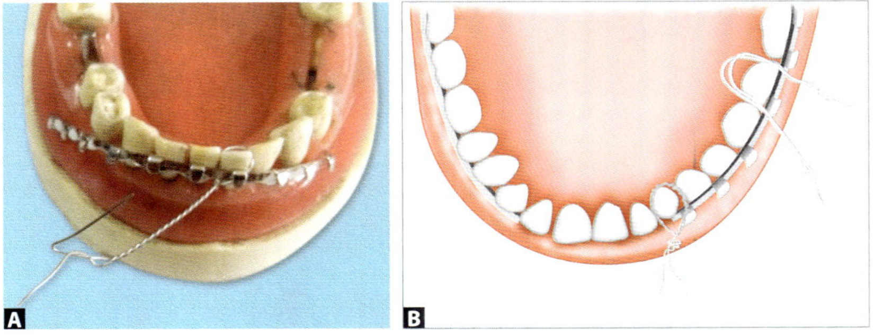

Figs 4A and B: Wire is twisted around the lug to get stable fixation of arch bar

- Similarly arch bar is tightened on adjacent tooth (Figs 5A and B).

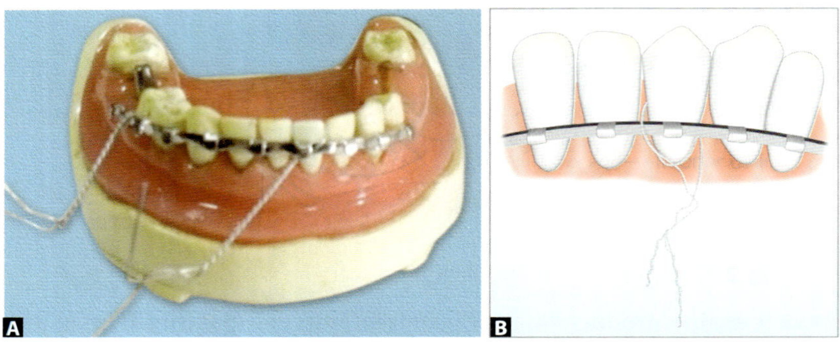

Figs 5A and B: Tightening around adjacent tooth

- Similarly arch bar is tightened on upper as well as lower dental arch (Figs 6A to C).

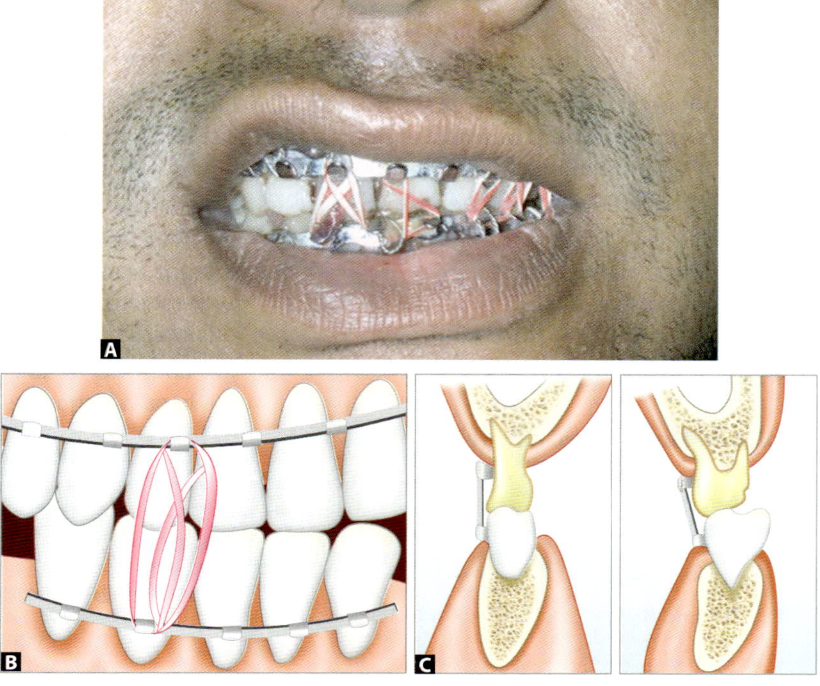

Figs 6A to C: Maxillomandibular fixation achieved through elastic bands/wires

WIRING TECHNIQUES

Gilmer Method

Advantages

- Simple technique
- Effective technique
- Do not require arch bars.

Disadvantages

- Fracture site cannot be inspected because of inability to open mouth. This can only be done after cutting the wire.

Steps

- **Infiltration**: Two percent lignocaine with adrenaline is injected at upper and lower gingivobuccal sulcus:
  - Mental nerve block given
  - Inferior alveolar nerve block given
- Twenty six number wire is introduced through interdental space labially and is retrieved on lingual side (Fig. 7).

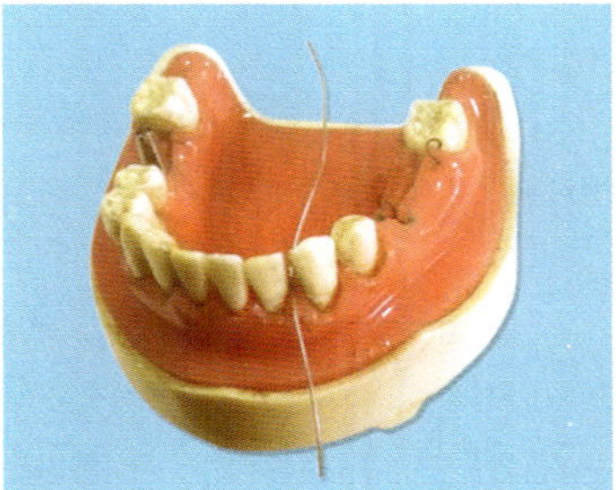

Fig. 7: Wire is passed from labial to lingual side through interdental space

- Wire is again introduced into adjacent interdental space from lingual side and retrieved again on labial side (Fig. 8).

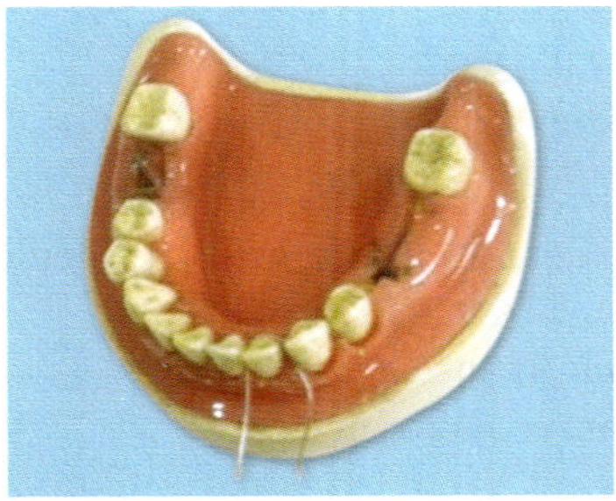

Fig. 8: Wire is retrieved from lingual to labial side through adjacent interdental space

- With the help of twister, the wire is twisted and tightened around neck of tooth (Figs 9A and B).

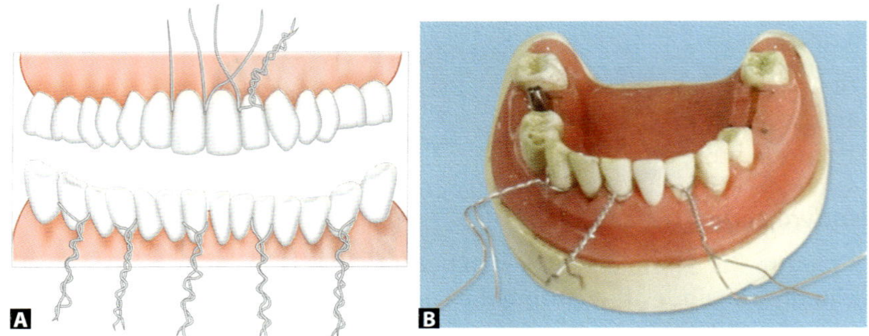

Figs 9A and B: Twisting of wire around neck of teeth

- Adequate number of wires are passed through upper and lower teeth
- The teeth are brought into occlusion and immobilized by twisting one upper and lower wire (Fig. 10).

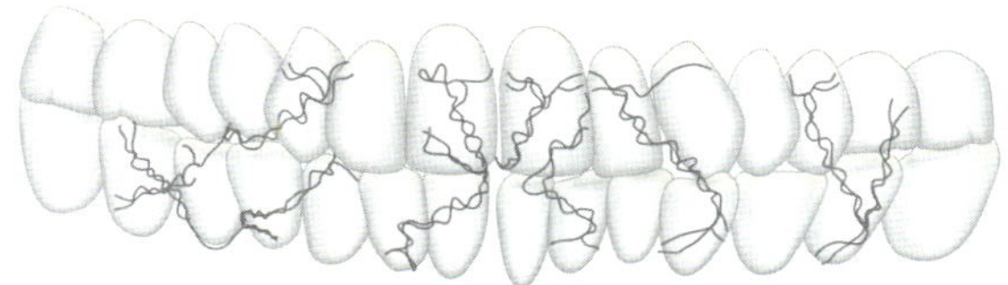

Fig. 10: Teeth in occlusion after maxillomandibular fixation

Eyelet Method

Advantages

- Simple and cost-effective technique
- It can be done without arch bar
- Fracture site can be inspected.

Disadvantages

- Chances of soft tissue injury
- Risk of blood-borne infections.

Steps

- **Infiltration:** Two percent lignocaine with adrenaline is injected at upper and lower gingivobuccal sulcus
  - Mental nerve block given
  - Inferior alveolar nerve block given
- Adequate size of around 20 cm wire is cut and looped around drill bit and twisted on drill bit for two and a half turns (Fig. 11).

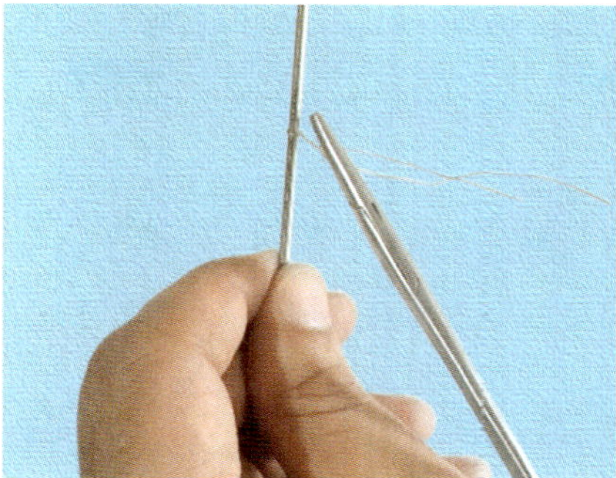

Fig. 11: Loop is made by twisting the wire around a drill bit by two and half turn

- This forms a loop at one end of a wire (Fig. 12).

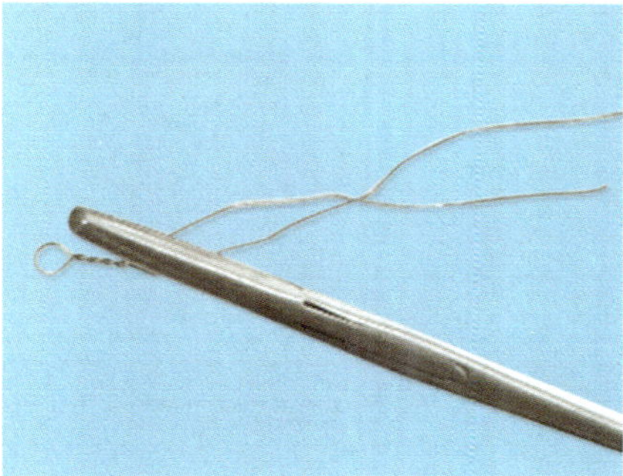

Fig. 12: Picture showing the loop

- Then other two ends of wire are passed through interdental space from buccal side and retrieved to the lingual side (Fig. 13).

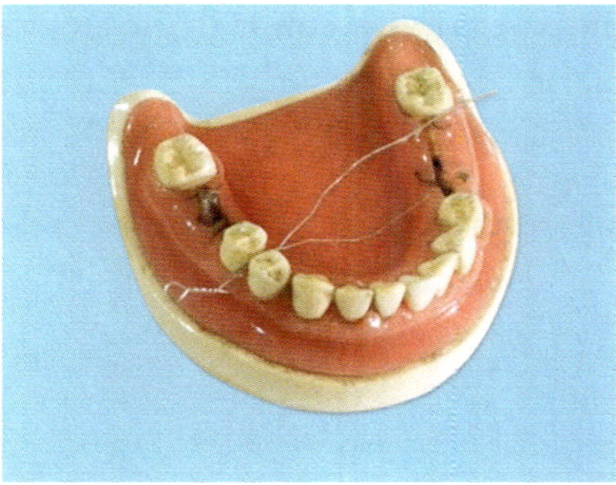

Fig. 13: Free ends of the wire are passed through interdental space from buccal to lingual side

- Then one end of wire is passed through posterior interdental space from lingual to buccal side (Fig. 14).

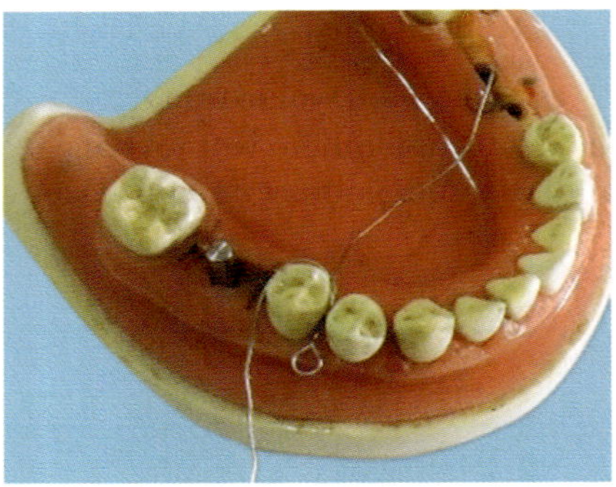

Fig. 14: One end of the wire is retrieved from lingual to buccal side through adjacent posterior interdental space

- Other end of wire is passed through anterior interdental space in the same manner (Fig. 15).

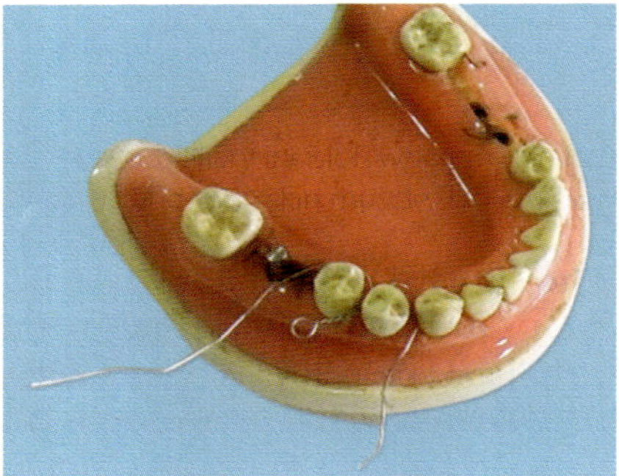

Fig. 15: Other end of the wire is retrieved from lingual to buccal side through adjacent anterior interdental space

- Then any end of the wire is passed through the loop (Fig. 16).

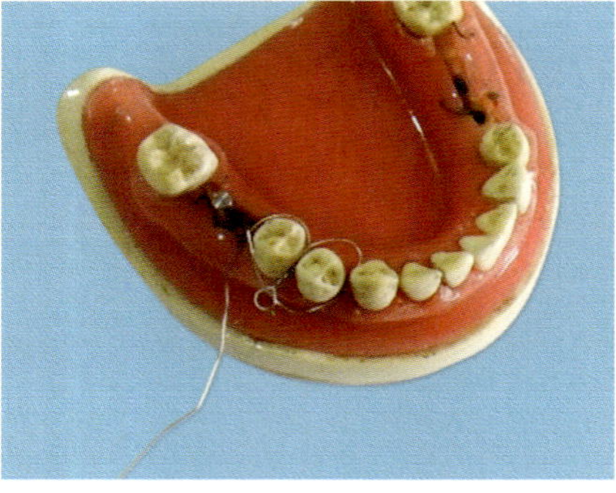

Fig. 16: One of the free end of wire is passed through the loop

- Free ends of both the wires are tightened around the tooth (Fig. 17).

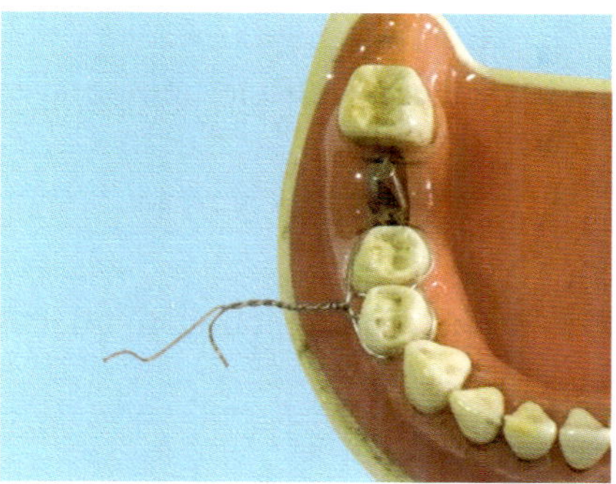

Fig. 17: Free ends of wire are twisted around the neck of the teeth

- Normally, the eyelet wires are placed around premolar tooth at four quadrants of oral cavity (Figs 18A and B).

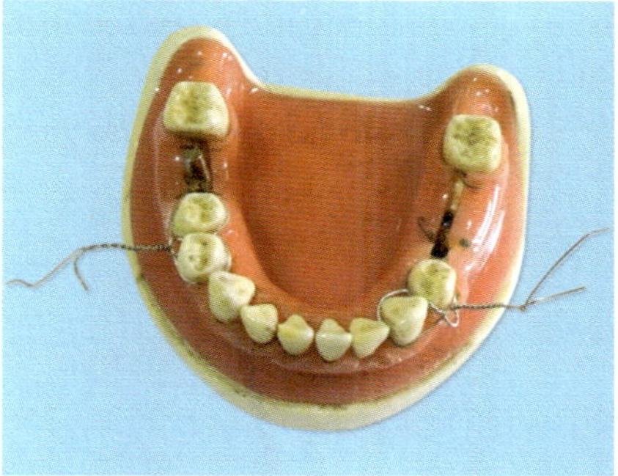

Fig. 18A: Similarly eyelets are passed through other premolars

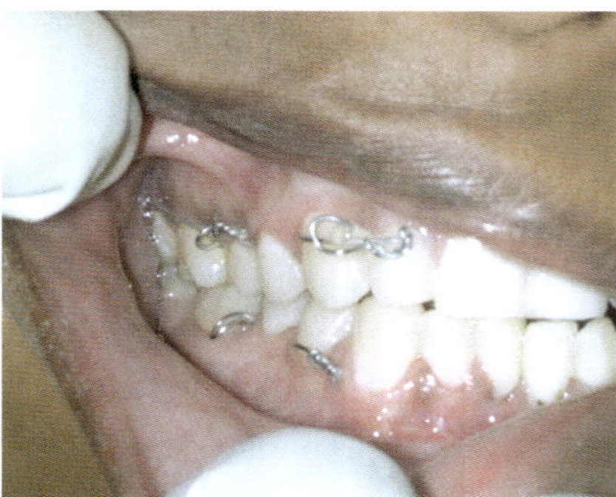

Figs 18B: Eyelets passed through upper and lower dental arch

- After achieving the occlusion, a wire is passed through upper and lower loop and is tightened for maxillomandibular fixation (MMF).

Ernst Ligature

Indications

- In case of emergencies, it can be used for temporary fixation prior to any definitive operative technique
- It can be used for simple fractures.

Disadvantages

- It cannot be used for unstable, comminuted or infected fractures
- It cannot be used around loose tooth
- Risk of blood-borne infections.

Steps

- **Infiltration:** Two percent lignocaine with adrenaline is injected at upper and lower gingivobuccal sulcus:
  - Mental nerve block given
  - Inferior alveolar nerve block given
- Adequate size (20 cm) of wire is cut and is passed through one interdental space from labial side to lingual side (Fig. 19).
- This wire is threaded back from adjacent anterior interdental space from lingual to labial side (Fig. 20).

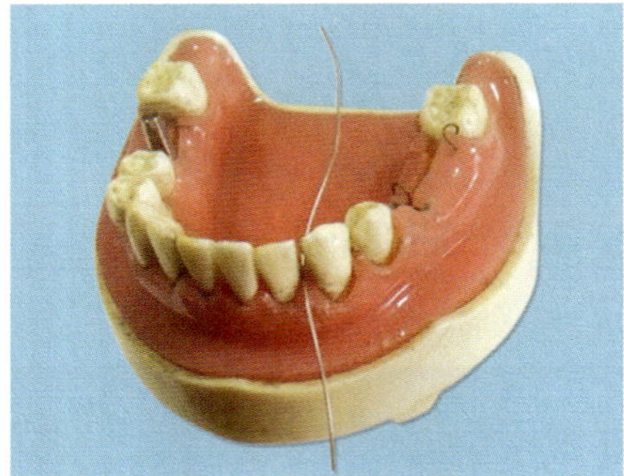

Fig. 19: Wire is passed through interdental space from labial to lingual side

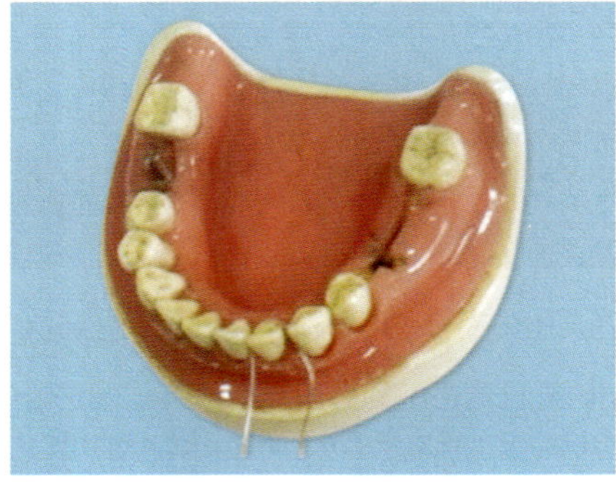

Fig. 20: Wire is again retrieved from lingual to labial side through adjacent interdental space

- The anterior end of the wire is passed from posterior interdental space from buccal to lingual side (Fig. 21).

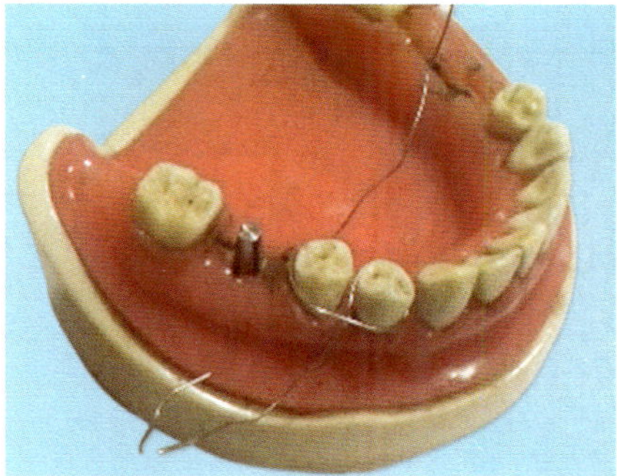

Fig. 21: The anterior free end of wire is passed from labial to lingual side through posterior interdental space

- This end of the wire is retrieved again on buccal side by passing through the adjacent anterior interdental space (Fig. 22).

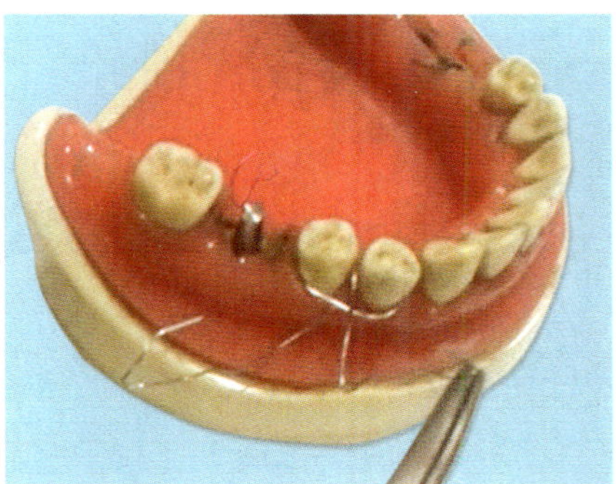

Fig. 22: Same end of wire is retrieved from lingual to labial side through adjacent interdental space

- This forms a loop around two teeth which is pulled and twisted (Fig. 23).

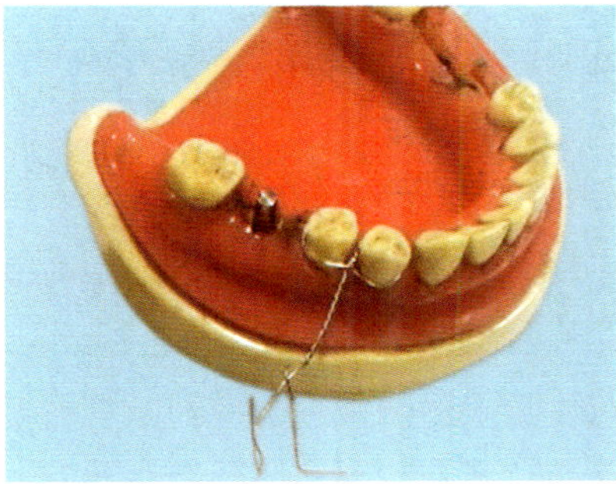

Fig. 23: Free end of the wire are twisted around neck of teeth

- This is normally done on premolar teeth
- Similar tightening is done on adjacent tooth (Fig. 24).

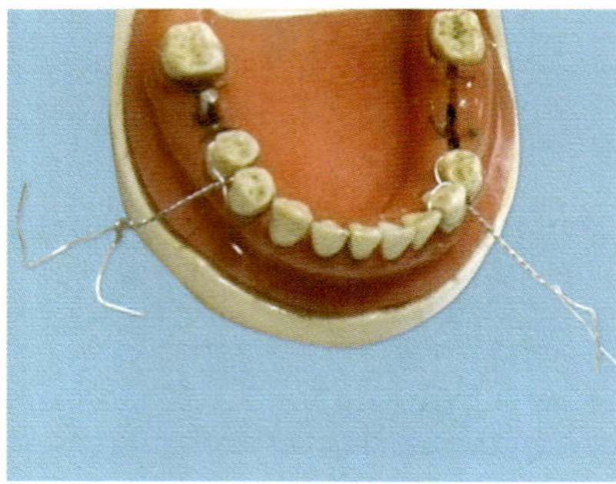

Fig. 24: Similar ligatures formed around other premolars

- Then upper and lower wire is twisted around each other to achieve maxillomandibular fixation.

INTERMAXILLARY SCREW FIXATION

Advantages

- Time saving technique
- Rapid method of immobilization
- Least chances of blood-borne infections
- Least chances of soft tissue injury.

Disadvantages

- Cost affair
- Requires precise placement
- Chances of damage to roots of mandibular or maxillary tooth
- It cannot be done on complicated and comminuted fractures
- Normally done in general anesthesia.

Steps

- These screws are readily available in market in standard sizes. These screws are inserted according to the type of fractures (Fig. 25).

- Screws are positioned in maxilla and mandible in such a way that roots of maxillary and mandibular tooth is not traumatized.

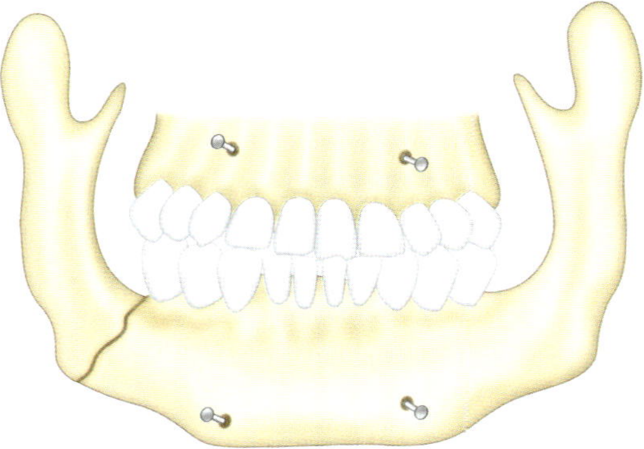

Fig. 25: Intermaxillary screws fixed on upper and lower alveolus

- These screws have preformed holes in it. Wire is passed through these preformed holes and fixation is accomplished (Fig. 26).

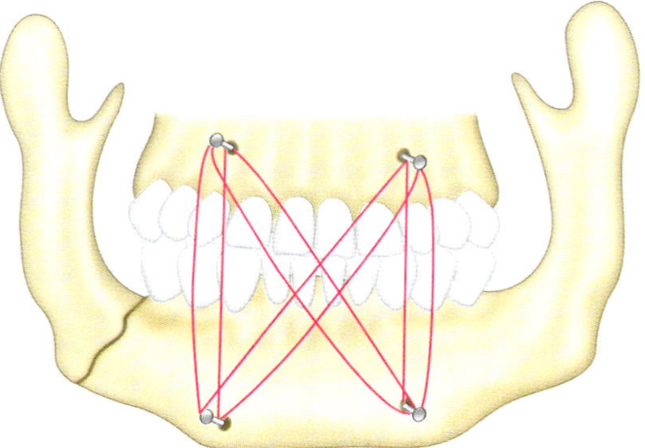

Fig. 26: Wires are passed through preformed holes in the intermaxillary screws to achieve maxillomandibular fixation

CHAPTER

Infiltration Techniques of Interest

LOCAL ANESTHESIA TECHNIQUES

- Intermaxillary fixation (IMF) is best done under local anesthesia if patient is cooperative hence intraoperative retraction is less resulting into minimal postoperative edema
- For doing IMF, both upper and lower jaws need to be anesthetized.

AREA OF INFILTRATION

Upper Jaw Infiltration

Anesthesia needed are:

1. Posterior superior alveolar nerve block.
2. Middle superior alveolar nerve block.
3. Anterior superior alveolar nerve block (infraorbital nerve block).
4. Greater palatine nerve block.
5. Incisive foramen nerve block.

Posterior Superior Alveolar Nerve Block

Goal

Goal is to deposit the local anesthesia close to the posterior superior alveolar (PSA) nerve located posterior superior and medial to the maxillary tuberosity (Fig. 1).

Area anesthetized are (Fig. 2):

- Maxillary 1st molar
- Maxillary 2nd molar
- Maxillary 3rd molar.

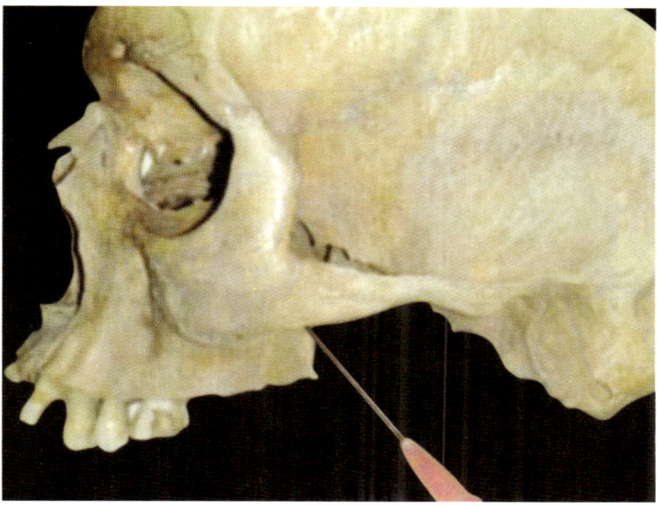

Fig. 1: Area where local anesthesia is deposited in posterior superior alveolar (PSA) nerve block

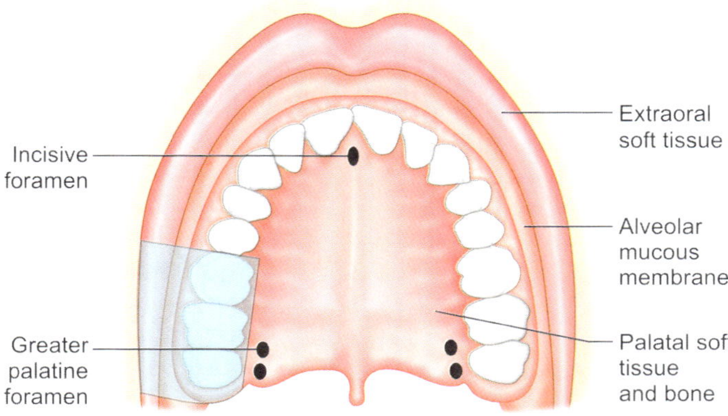

Fig. 2: Area anesthetized by anterior superior alveolar nerve block

Steps

Twenty six number short needle is used:

- Orient the bevel end of the needle towards bone
- Partially open the patient's mouth, pulling the mandible to the side of injection
- Retract the patient's cheek with your finger
- Insert the needle into a height of mucobuccal fold over second molar (Fig. 3)

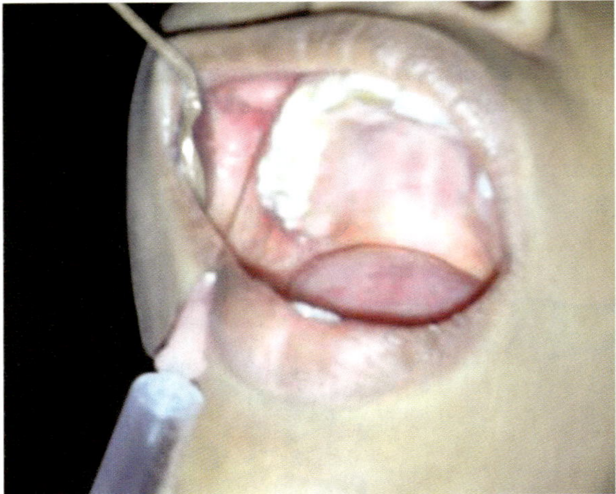

Fig. 3: Area of infiltration

- Advance the needle slowly in upward, inward and backward direction
- Slowly advance to the soft tissue
- If resistance is felt, withdraw the needle slightly and change the direction and re-advance again.

Middle Superior Alveolar Nerve Block (Fig. 4)

Goals

Deposition of anesthesia above the maxillary 2nd premolar.

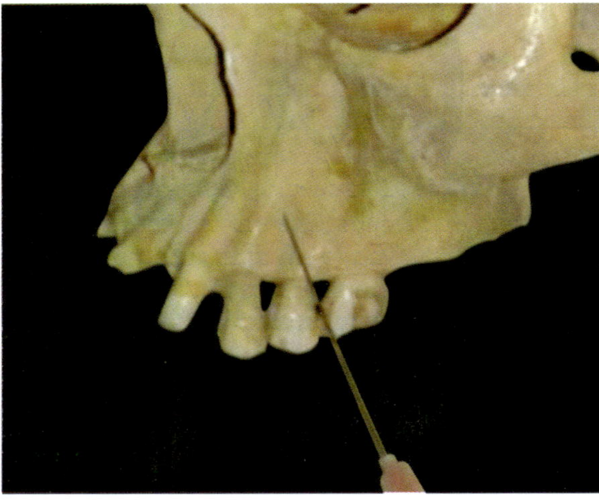

Fig. 4: Area where local anesthesia is deposited for middle superior alveolar nerve block

Areas anesthetized are (Fig. 5):

- Maxillary 1st premolar
- Maxillary 2nd premolar
- Partly maxillary 1st molar.

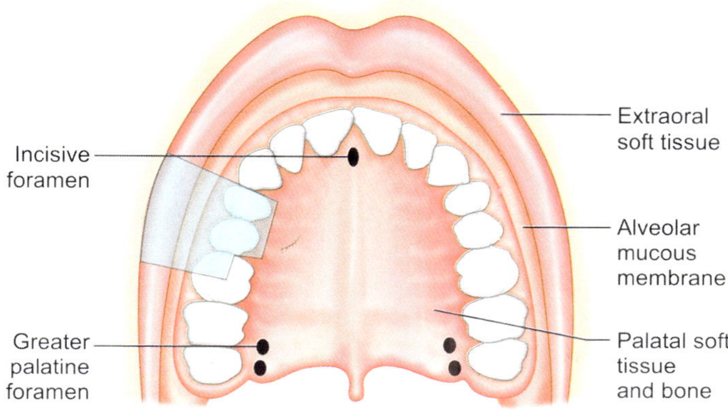

Fig. 5: Area anesthetized by middle superior alveolar nerve block

Technique

Twenty six number short needle used:

- Area of insertion, height of mucobuccal fold above the second premolar tooth (Fig. 6)

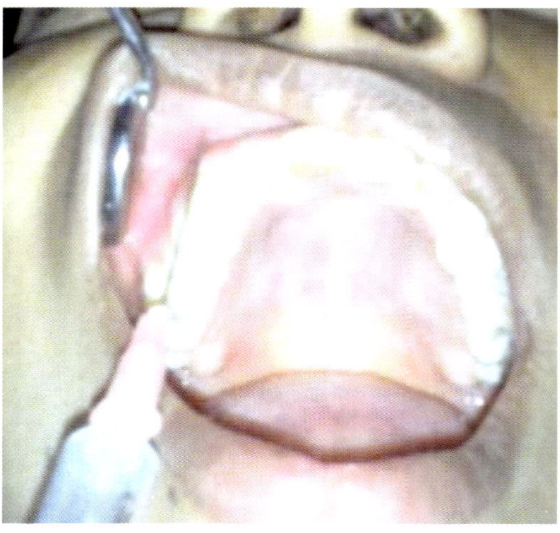

Fig. 6: Area from where anesthesia is injected

- Aspirate and if no blood then deposit 0.9–1 mL solution.

Anterior Superior Alveolar Nerve Block (Infraorbital Nerve Block)

Goal

Local anesthesia is deposited near infraorbital foramen (Fig. 7).

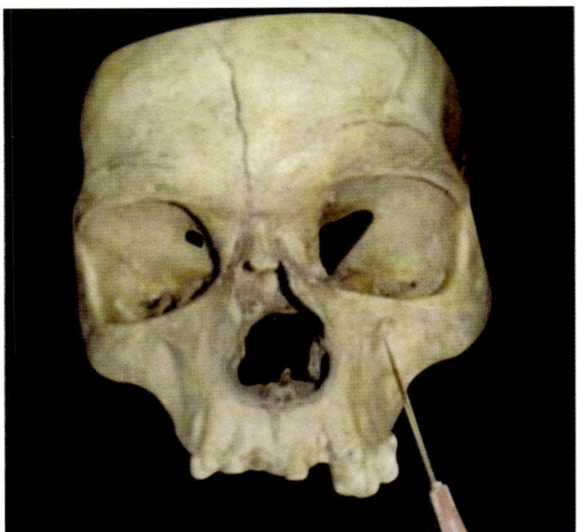

Fig. 7: Area where local anesthesia is deposited

Area anesthetized are (Fig. 8):

- Maxillary incisors
- Maxillary premolars
- Maxillary 1st molar.

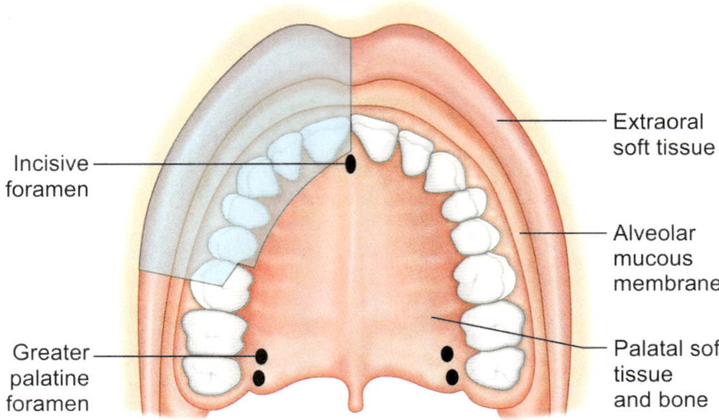

Fig. 8: Area anesthetized by anterior superior alveolar nerve block

Technique

- Target area—infraorbital foramen (below the infraorbital notch) (Fig. 9)
- Landmark—mucobuccal fold, infraorbital notch, infraorbital foramen
- Area of insertion—height of mucobuccal fold directly over first premolar.

Procedure

- Feel for infraorbital notch
- Move your fingers downward from the notch applying gentle pressure to the tissue.

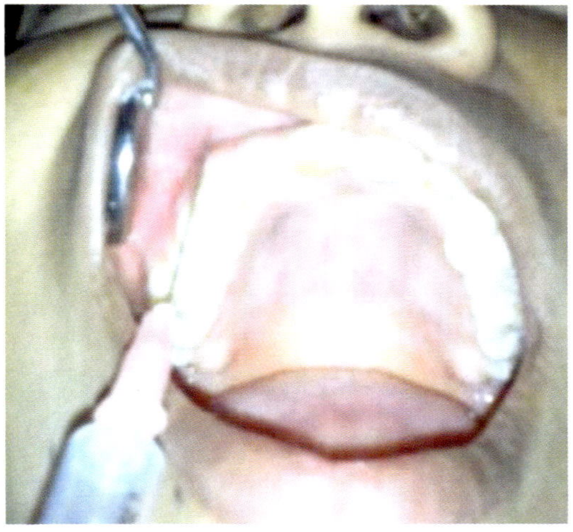

Fig. 9: Area where local anesthesia is injected for infraorbital block

The bone immediately inferior to the notch is convex, this represents the lower border of orbit and a roof of infraorbital foramen:

- As your finger continues, inferiorly a concavity is felt, this is infraorbital foramen
- Maintain your finger on the foramen or mark the skin at the site
- Retract the lips, pull the tissue in mucobuccal fold
- Insert the needle into the height of mucobuccal fold over the first premolar with the bevel facing bone
- Reach to the required site and deposit the local anesthetic agent.

Greater Palatine Nerve Block

Goals

Deposition of anesthesia at greater palatine foramen.

Areas anesthetized are (Fig. 10):

- Posterior portion of hard palate

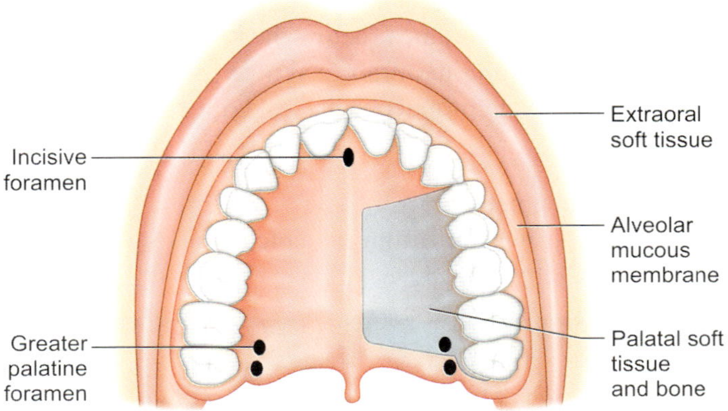

Fig. 10: Area which is blocked by greater palatine block

- Target area—greater palatine nerve as it passes anteriorly between the soft tissue and bone of the heart palate
- Landmark—junction of maxillary alveolar process and palatine bone
- Part of insertion—advance the syringe from the opposite side of the mouth at the right angle to the target area.

Procedure

- Feel for depression of greater palatine foramen with the help of cotton swab and a finger (Fig. 11)
- The foramen is located distal to second molar, but it may be either anterior or posterior to its usual position
- Inject in the foramen area around few drops.

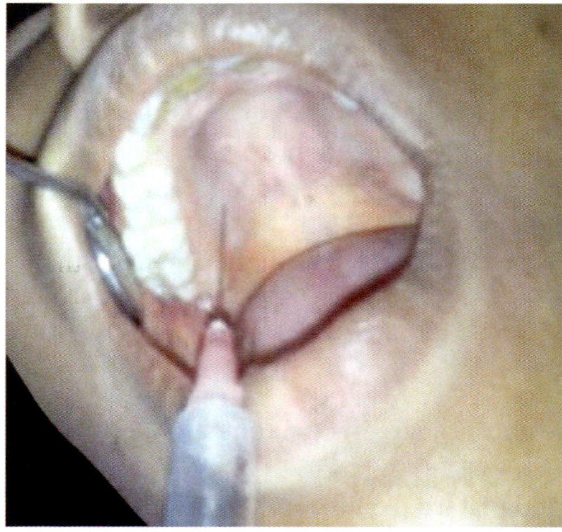

Fig. 11: Area where greater palatine foramen is located

Lower Jaw Infiltration

1 Inferior alveolar nerve block
2. Mental nerve block.

Inferior Alveolar Nerve Block (Mandibular Nerve Block)

Goals

Deposition of anesthesia near inferior alveolar nerve (Fig. 12).

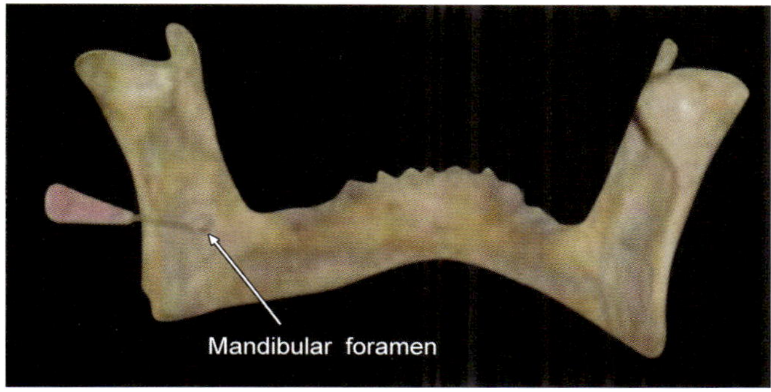

Fig. 12: Area where infra-alveolar nerve is located

Area anesthetized are (Fig. 13):
- Mandibular teeth to the midline
- Body and part of ramus
- Part of tongue and floor of mouth.

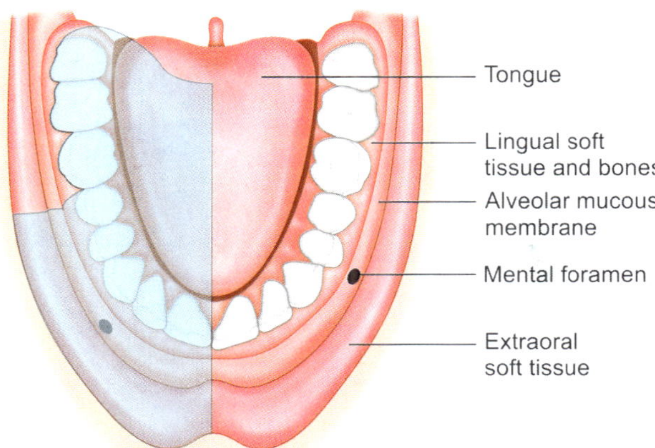

Fig. 13: Area anesthesized by infra-alveolar nerve block

Procedure

- A fingertip is kept in the coronoid notch
- An imaginary line extended posterior from the fingertip in the coronoid notch to the deepest part of the pterygomandibular raphe
- This imaginary line should be parallel with the occlusal plane of the mandibular molar teeth
- The needle is inserted at anteroposterior distance from the coronoid notch back to the deepest part of the pterygomandibular raphe (Fig. 14)

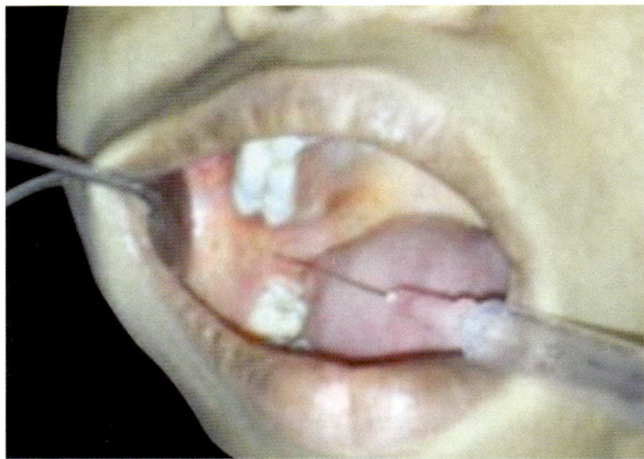

Fig. 14: Area where anesthesia is given

- The finger in the coronoid notch is used to pull the tissue laterally, stretching them over the injection side making them taut for better visibility and less traumatic.

Mental Nerve Block

Goal

Local anesthesia is deposited at mental foramen (Fig. 15).

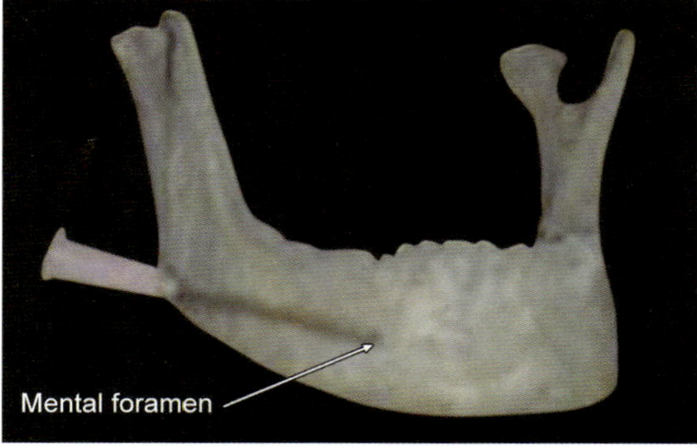

Fig. 15: Location of mental foramen

Area anesthetized are (Fig. 16)

- Soft tissue lying anterior to the foramen
- Soft tissue of lower lip and chin at the site of injection.

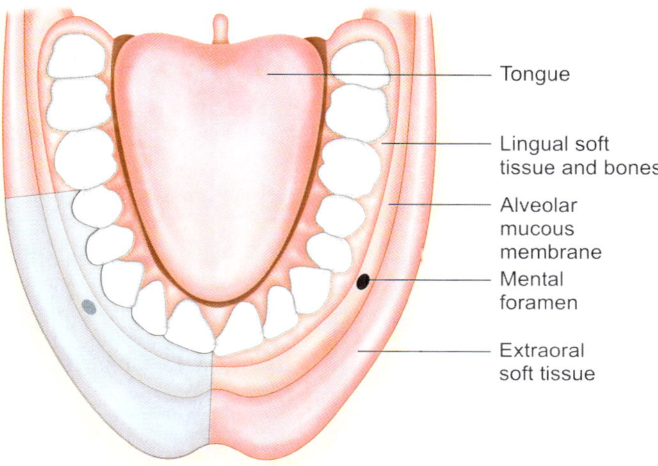

Fig. 16: Area anesthetized by mental nerve block

Procedure

- A 24-gauge needle with 1 inch length is inserted in mucolabial fold in between two premolar directing downward and anteriorly after retracting the cheek (Fig. 17).

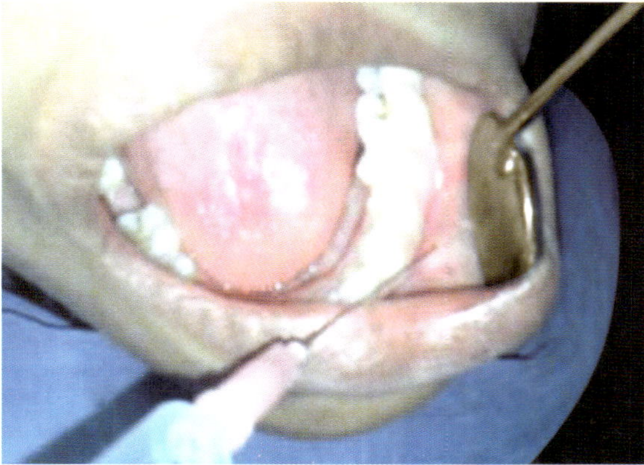

Fig. 17: Area in which local anesthesia is injected for mental nerve block

- It contacts the bone at the level of apex at the second premolar anterior to it
- After aspiration, 0.5 mL of local agent is slowly injected.

Approaches to Mandibular Fracture

The mandible is involved in 70% of patients with facial fractures. It is the second commonest fracture after nasal bone fractures.

FREQUENCY OF THE FRACTURE (FIG. 1)

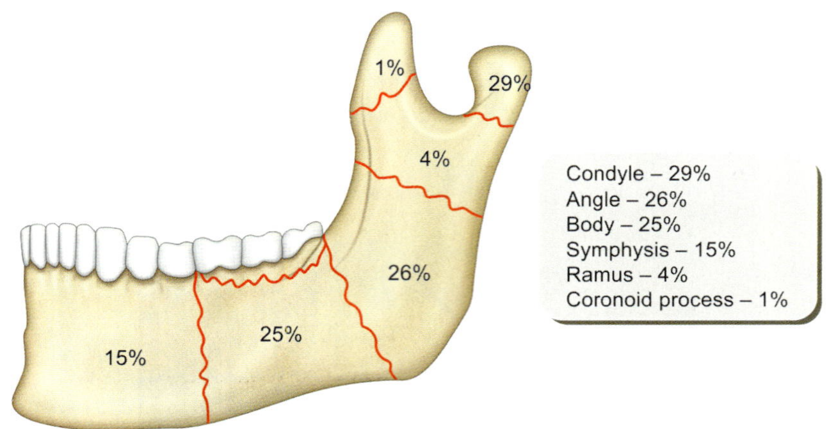

Fig. 1: Frequency of mandiblar fracture according to location

APPROACHES TO SYMPHYSIS AND PARASYMPHYSIS FRACTURES

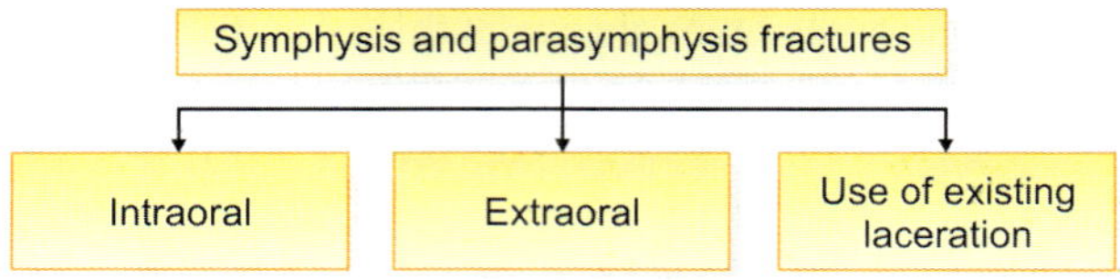

Intraoral Approach

Indications

All simple symphysis and parasymphysis fractures.

Advantages

- No visible scar
- Incision can be extended posterioly in cases of angle and body fractures.

Disadvantage

In complex/comminuted/infected/edentulous symphyseal and parasymphyseal fractures where large area of exposure is required for placement of load bearing osteosynthesis. Extraoral incision is preferred in such cases.

Infilteration

Inject the site with 2% xylocaine and adrenaline (1:200,000), and wait for few minutes.

Incision

- Incision is made all along the gingivolabial sulcus at symphysis and parasymphysis area (between two canines) few millimeters away from the attached margin (Figs 2A and B).
- Incision can be taken by 15 number blade or by electrocautery.

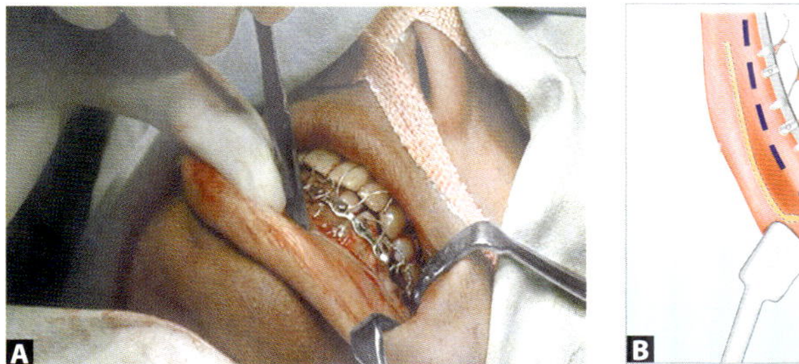

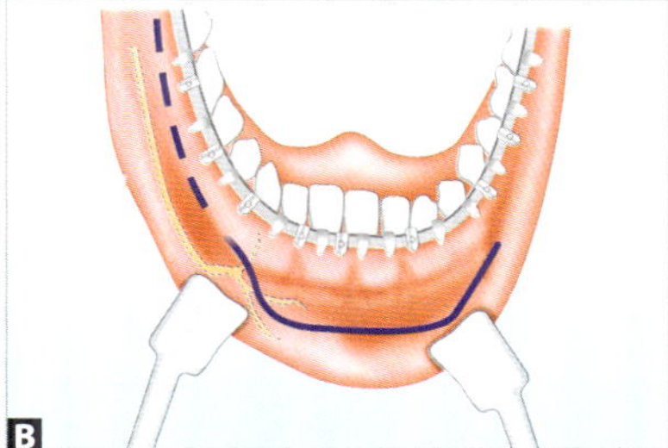

Figs 2A and 2B: Incision is taken 5 mm away from the gingivobuccal sulcus

- Dissection is further continued through the mentalis muscle (Figs 3A and B).

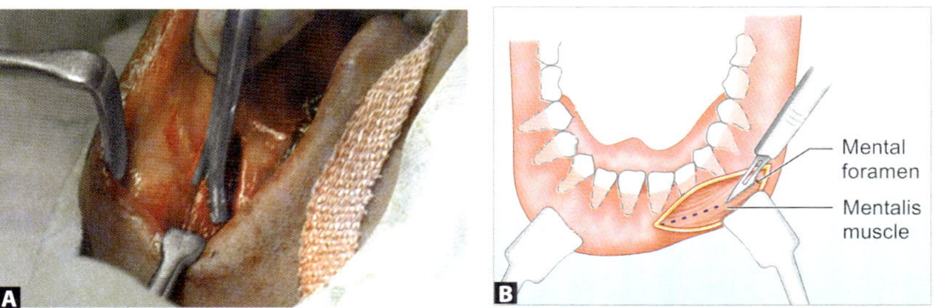

Figs 3A and B: Dissection through mentalis muscle

- Utmost care should be taken to delineate and preserve branches of mental nerve (Figs 4A and B).

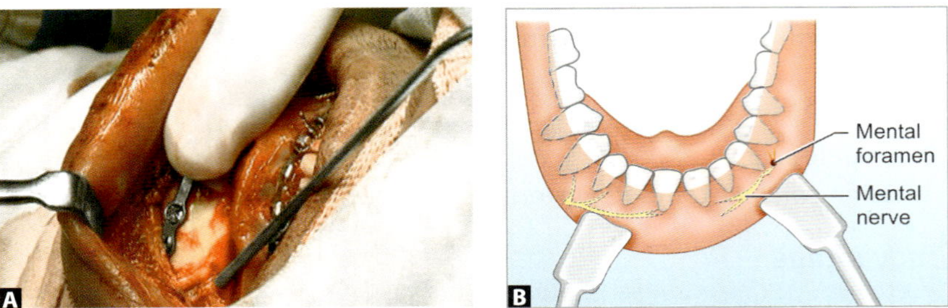

Figs 4A and B: Preservation of mental nerve

- Adequate stump of muscle should be preserved on either sides so that suturing of muscle is not difficult.

Wound Closure

After a thorough betadine wash, wound is closed in layers. Mentalis muscle is reapproximated to prevent drooping of chin tissue. Mucosal layer is sutured in a simple interrupted fashion (Figs 5A and B).

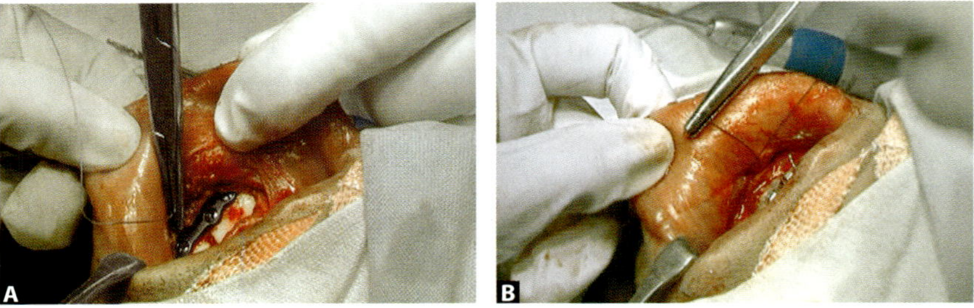

Figs 5A and B: (A) Showing closure of muscle layer; (B) Showing closure of mucosal layer

Extraoral Approach

Indications

For complex/comminuted/infected/edentulous symphyseal and parasymphyseal fractures where large area of exposure is required for placement of load bearing osteosynthesis.

Advantages

- No major neurovascular structure present in this area
- Lingual surface of the mandible can be easily inspected to assure optimum reduction of fracture in this segment.

Incision

- The incision will follow the normal curvature of the anterior mandible (Fig. 6).
- Incision has to taken in the normal skin crease.

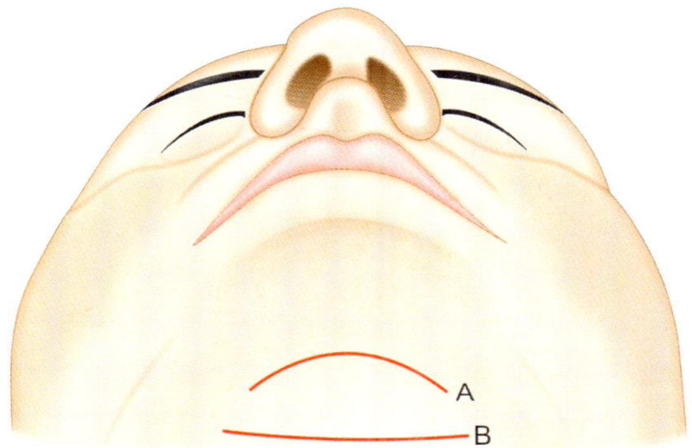

Fig. 6: Variations in incision: (A) Following curvature of anterior mandible; (B) Hidden in submental skin crease

Infiltration

Incision area is infilterated with 2% lignocaine + adrenaline.

Dissection

- Skin and subcutaneous layer incised with subplatysmal flaps elevated staying close to the curvature of the mandible
- Mylohyoid muscle need not to be dissected
- Palpate the mandible and skeletonize the anterior border of mandible with the help of a cautery
- Further dissection is carried according to the fracture site.

Wound Closure

Wound is closed in the following order:

a. Muscle layer
b. Platysmal layer
c. Skin

Surgical Dressing

A crepe bandage dressing (Fig. 7) is given to:

- Eliminate dead space
- Prevent hematoma formation
- Support soft tissues in place.

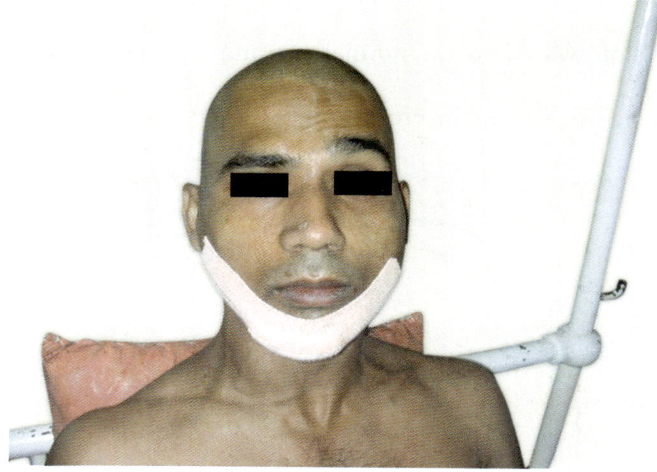

Fig. 7: Crepe bandage pressure dressing

USE OF EXISTING LACERATION

Advantage

No new incision is required (Fig. 8).

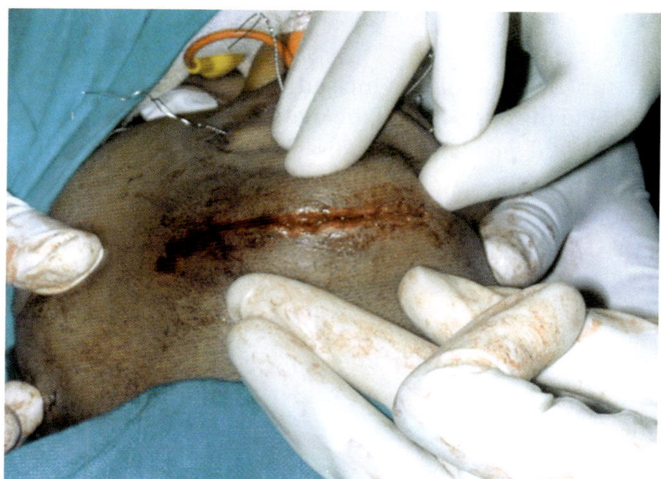

Fig. 8: Preexisting laceration wound in a case of parashymphysis fracture

Dissection

The existing wound can be extrapolated for the management of fracture. The same incision can be extended for further access to the fracture site as per requirement (Fig. 9).

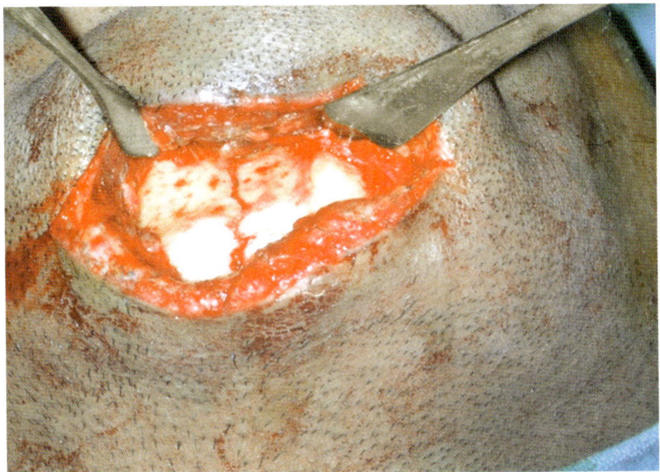

Fig. 9: Dissection through the same wound to expose the fracture site

Wound Closure

Primary closure is done in layers after achieving proper hemostasis and thorough saline and betadine wash several times.

Note: Simple symphysis and parasymphysis fractures with minimal displacement can be managed under local anesthesia.

In cases of complex/comminuted/infected/edentulous/malunion or nonunion cases, general anesthesia is preferred.

APPROACHES TO BODY AND ANGLE

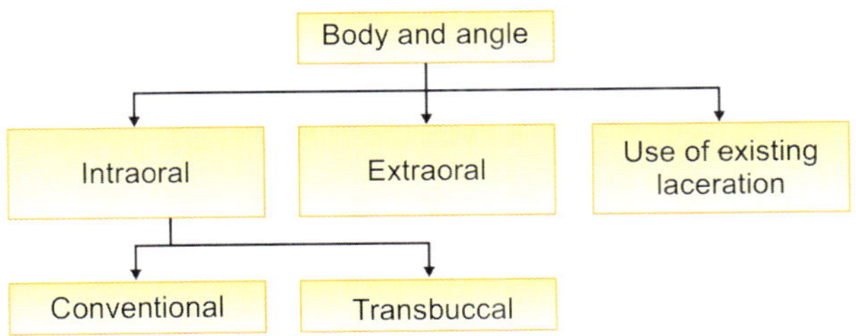

Intraoral

Conventional Approach

Indication

All simple angle and body fractures.

Advantages

- No visible scar
- Less morbidity and less hospital stay.

Disadvantages

- Restricted area for surgical manipulation
- In complex/comminuted/infected fractures where large area of exposure is required for placement of load bearing osteosynthesis, extraoral incision is preferred.

Infiltration

Inject the site with 2% xylocaine and adrenaline (1:200,000), and wait for few minutes.

Incision

- Incision varies upon the presence of 3rd molar in the fracture line
- If the 3rd molar needs to be removed then incision is made along the attached gingivobuccal sulcus of the molar tooth (Fig. 10A)

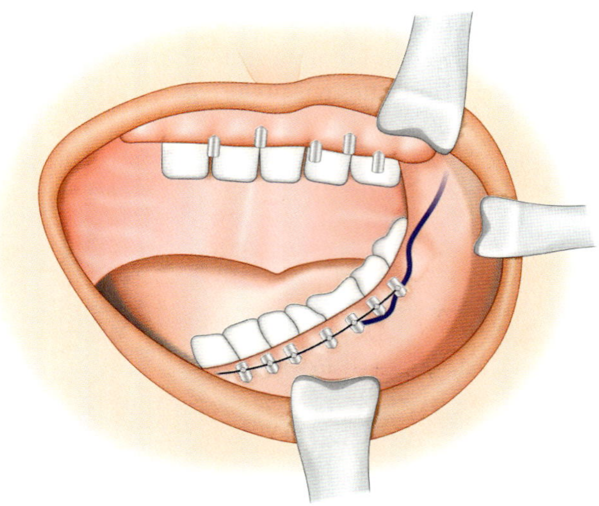

Fig. 10A: Incision along the gingivobuccal sulcus (3rd molar needs to be removed)

- Where in incision is taken 5 mm away from the attached surface of gingivobuccal sulcus when extraction is not required (Fig. 10B).

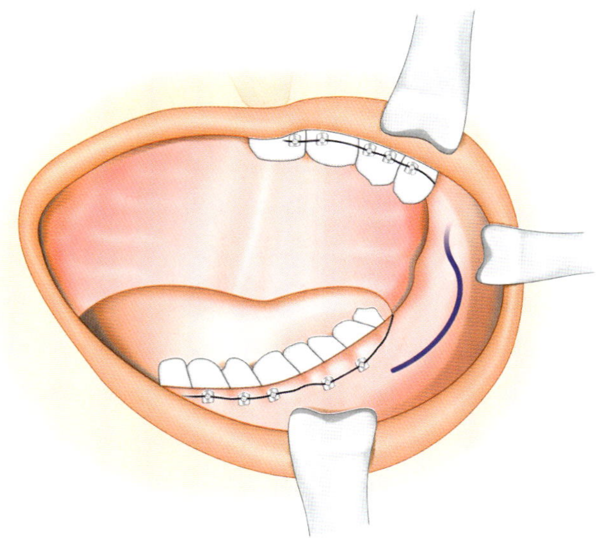

Fig. 10B: Incision 5 mm away from the attached margin of gingivobuccal sulcus (3rd molar needs to be retained)

- Incision line is drawn with the help of a surgical marker as per the presence of 3rd molar described above.

Dissection

Dissection is done along the incision line with the help of an electrocautery. This dissection is further deepened through the lower attachment of buccinator muscle to skeletonize the angle and body till the external oblique ridge (Figs 11A and B).

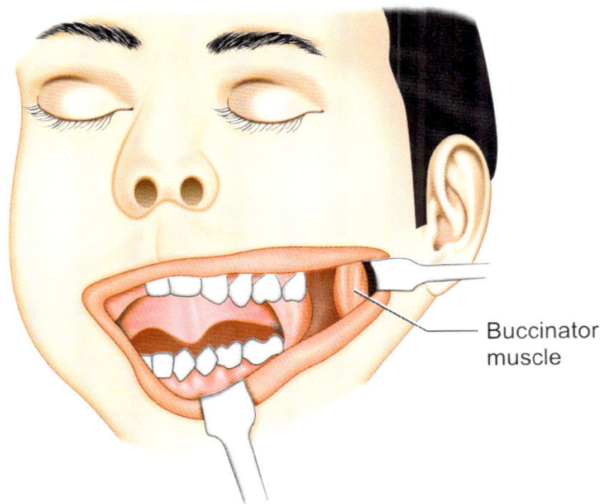

Fig. 11A: Lower attachment of buccinator muscle is exposed

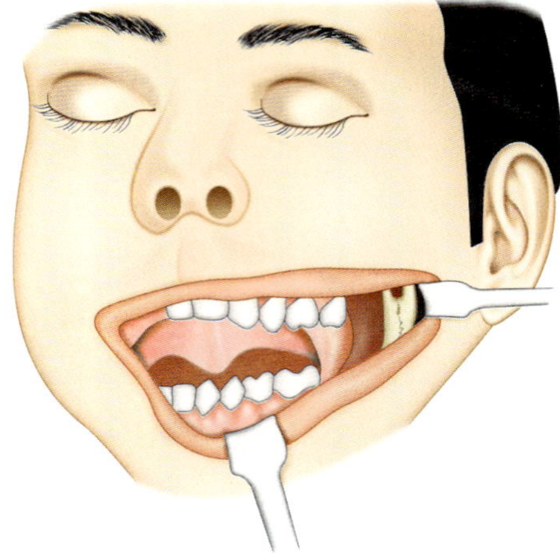

Fig. 11B: Buccinator muscle detached to expose fracture site

Precaution

The sensory buccal nerve crosses the upper anterior rim of ascending ramus of the mandible in the region of coronoid notch so a sharp dissection should be avoided at the posterior extension of the incision (as soon as lower coronoid notch is reached).

Wound Closure

After reduction and fixation of the fracture segment, wound is closed in layers. Utmost care should be taken that buccinator muscle is resutured to the cut stump.

Transbuccal System Approach

Advantages

This approach increases the versatility of transoral approach. Areas which are difficult to access with transoral approach can be easily accessed with this approach.

Disadvantages

- Special sets of instrument required
- Increased cost of the procedure.

Infiltration

Inject the site with 2% xylocaine and adrenaline (1:200,000), and wait for few minutes.

Incision

- Incision varies upon the presence of 3rd molar in the fracture line. If the 3rd molar needs to be removed then incision is made along the attached gingivobuccal sulcus of the molar tooth wherein incision is taken 5 mm away from the attached surface of gingivobuccal sulcus when extraction is not required (Fig. 12).

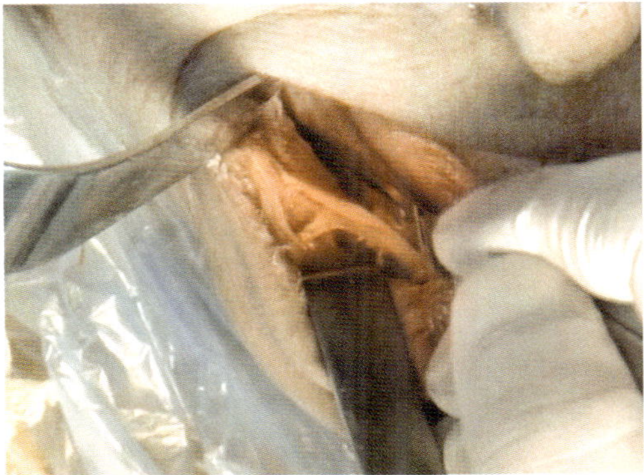

Fig. 12: Intraoral incision depending upon the presence of 3rd molar

Dissection

- Dissection is done along the incision line with the help of an electrocautery. This dissection is further deepened through the lower attachment of buccinator muscle to skeletonize the angle and body till the external oblique ridge (Fig. 13).

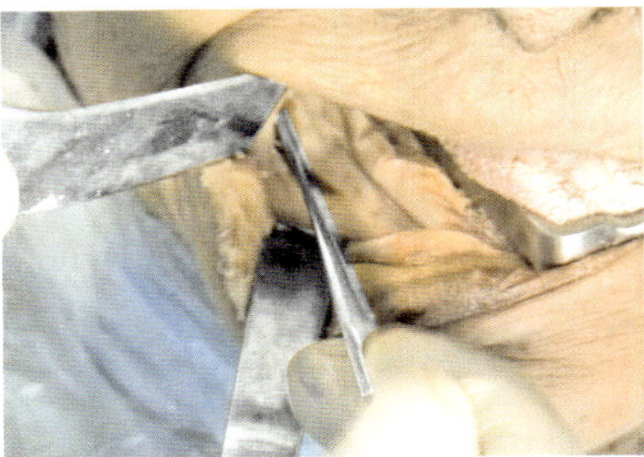

Fig. 13: Dissection carried till fracture site is exposed

Transbuccal System

- A small stab incision is made on the face. This stab incision is determined by the site of osteosynthesis or fracture site.
- This incision is normally taken in one of natural skin crease of the face. Incision should be parallel to the relaxed skin tension line (Fig. 14A).

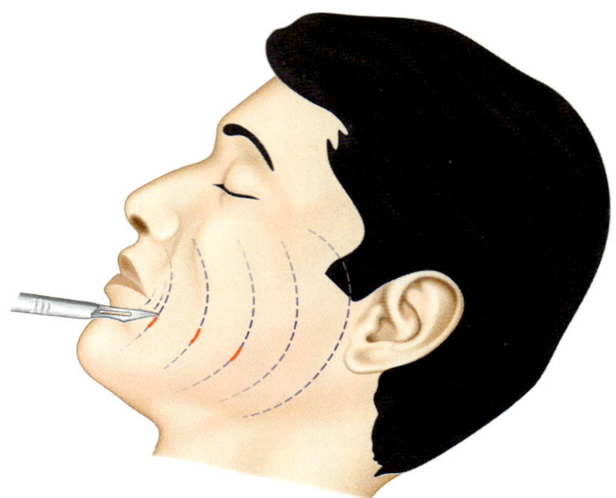

Fig. 14A: Incision along relaxed skin tension lines

- Through this incision, a trochar and cannula (Figs 14B and B) is inserted till the fracture site is reached.

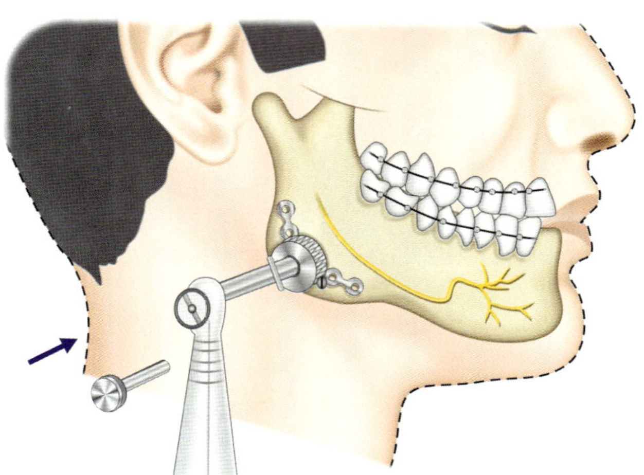

Fig. 14B

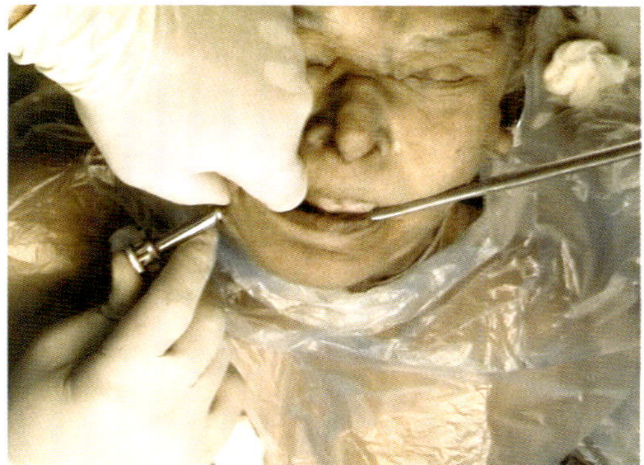

Fig. 14C

Figs 14B and C: Insertion of trochar and canrula at the fracture site

- Now the trochar is withdrawn and according to the need various retractors can be applied (Fig. 15).

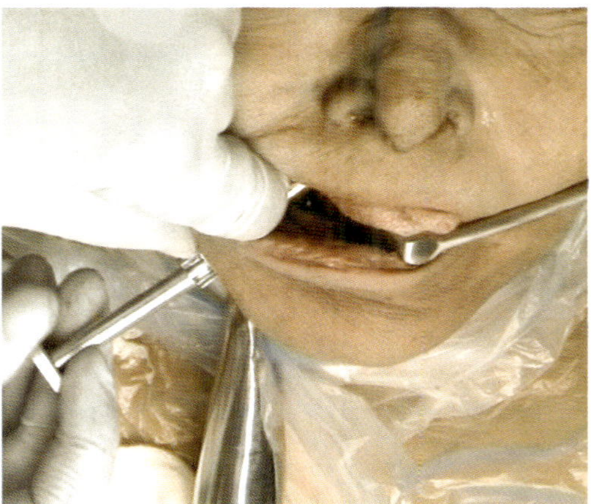

Fig. 15: Retractors applied to expose the fracture site

- Plate is then placed intraorally over the determined site (Fig. 16).

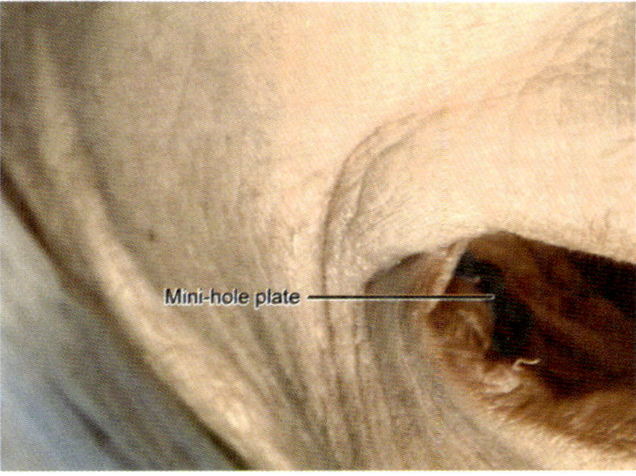

Fig. 16: Miniplate placed intraorally at the site of fracture

- Adequate size of drill bit is inserted through the cannula and required size of hole is made in the bone (Figs 17A and B).

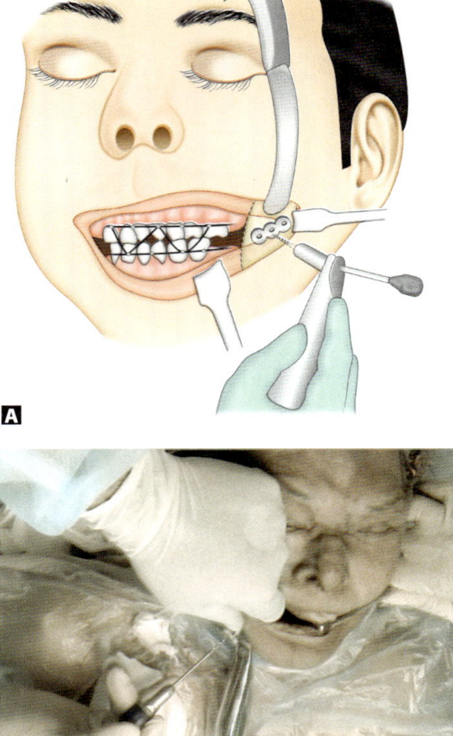

Figs 17A and B: Use of drill bits for making appropriate holes through the plate

- Through this cannula, screw is inserted using a self-holding screw driver (Fig. 18). In this way, adequate number of screws are inserted to secure the plate in place.

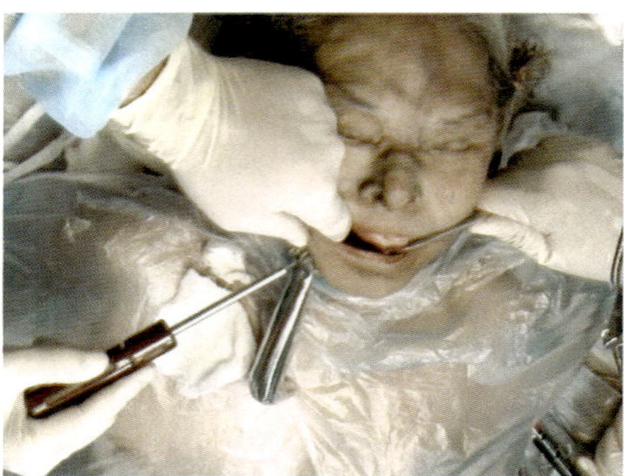

Fig. 18: Self-holding screw driver is used through cannula to fix required number of screws

- Then this transbuccal system is dismantled.

Extraoral Approach

Submandibular Approach (Risdon Approach)

Indications

Cases unsuitable for intraoral approaches such as complex/comminuted/ infected fractures where large area of exposure is required for placement of load wearing osteosynthesis.

Advantages

Large area of exposure for manipulation.

Disadvantages

- Visible scar
- Chances of injury to marginal mandibular nerve.

Infiltration

Incision

Incision is taken 2 finger breadth below the lower margin of the mandible or in a lower skin crease (Figs 19A and B).

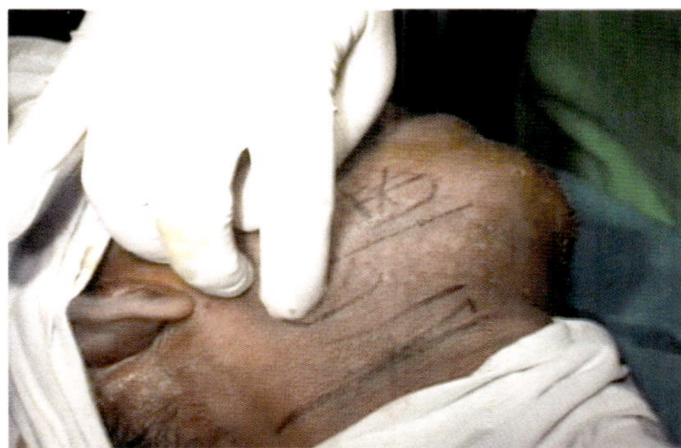

Fig. 19A: Marking of incision

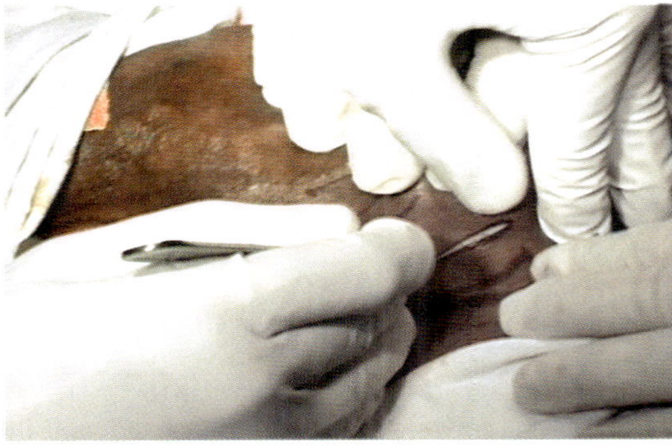

Fig. 19B: Placing the incision

Precautions

Utmost care should be taken to prevent any injury to the marginal mandibular nerve.

Various Methods to Prevent Injury to the Nerve

1. Without Identification of the Nerve

a. Dissection is strictly carried out in subplatysmal plane (Fig. 19C)

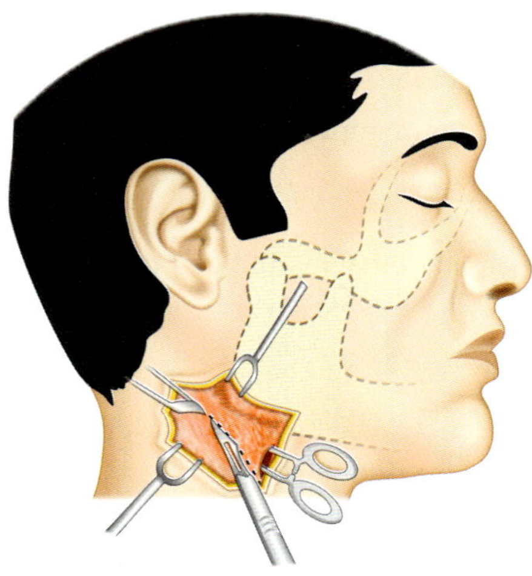

Fig. 19C: Elevation of subplatysmal flaps

- At the angle of mandible try to see the pulsation of facial artery and dissection is then carried out to skeletonize the facial vessels which is then ligated and retracted upwards (Fig. 19D).
- After doing this maneuver, nerve is automatically lifted up as it passes superficial to the facial vessels (**Hey's Martin method**)

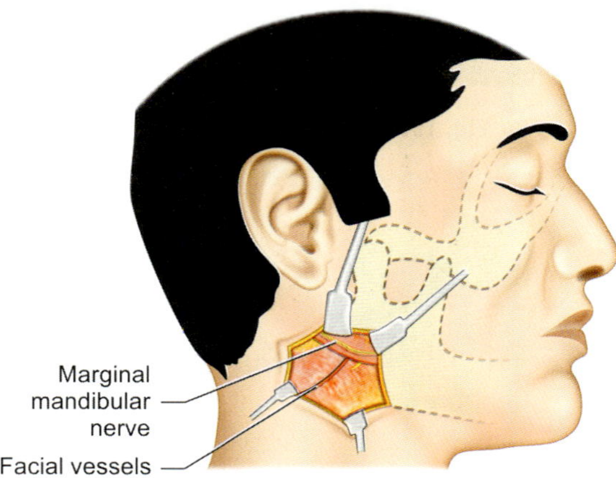

Fig. 19D: Marginal mandibular nerve passes superficial to facial vessels. Ligation and retraction of the vessels will automatically lift the nerve along with them (Hey's Martin method)

b. Dissection is carried out in deep cervical plane so that nerve is retracted in the flap without identifying it.

2. With Identification of the Nerve

a. Nerve is identified at the point 1 cm anteroinferior to the angle of mandible (Fig. 19E).
b. Nerve is identified superficial to external jugular vein at the point of its exit from parotid gland.

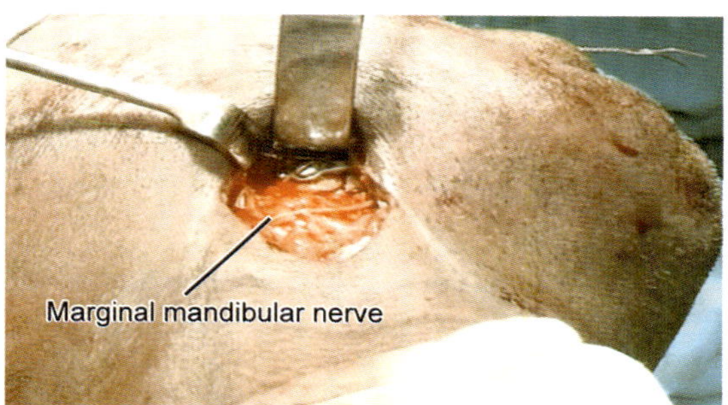

Fig. 19E: Identification of marginal mandibular nerve

- Further dissection is carried out till the lower border of mandible is identified. Massetor muscle is then cut and periosteal flap is elevated to expose the fracture site and external oblique ridge. Proper reduction and fixation is done after that.

Wound Closure

Wound is closed in layers in the following order (Fig. 19F):
- Muscle and periosteal layer
- Platysmal layer
- Skin

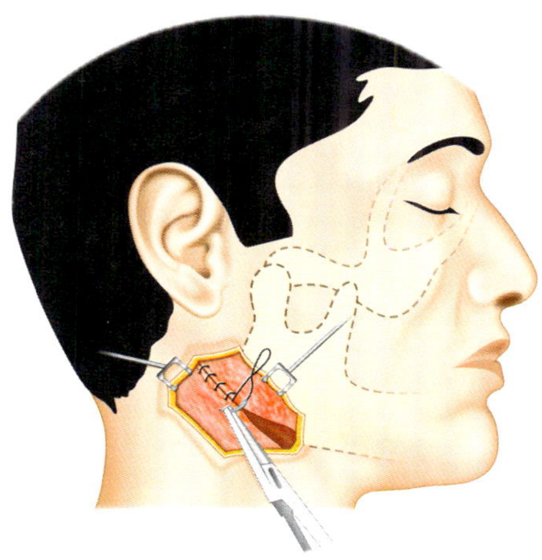

Fig. 19F: Closure of wound

Complications

- Bleeding
- Hematoma formation
- Injury to marginal mandibular nerve
- Wound dehiscence.

APPROACHES TO CONDYLAR AND SUBCONDYLAR FRACTURE

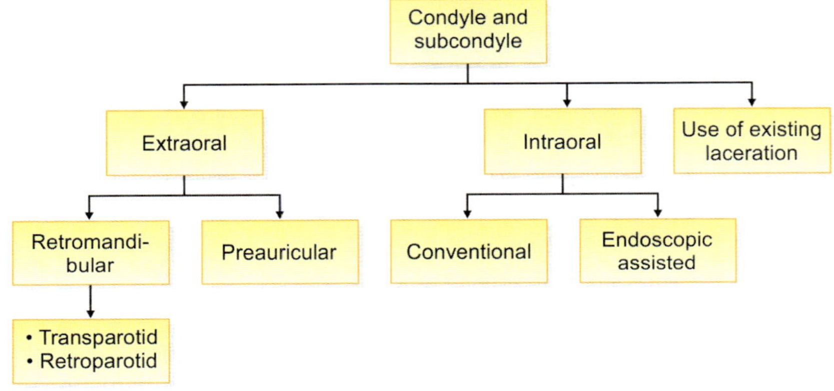

1. Extraoral
   A. Retromandibular
      - Transparotid
      - Retroparotid
   B. Preauricular
2. Intraoral
   A. Conventional
   B. Endoscopic assisted
3. Use of existing laceration

Retromandibular Approach

Retromandibular approach was first described by Hinds and Girotti in 1967. It was later on modified by Koberg and Momma in 1978. Hinds described it for the correction of mandibular prognathism.

Area Accessed

- Ramus
- Subcondyle
- Lower condyle fractures
- TM joint.

Incision

Incision begins 0.5 cm below the lobe of ear and continued inferiorly for 3–3.5 cm (Figs 20A and B). This incision is placed just behind the posterior border of mandible. Incision is not extended beyond angle of mandible.

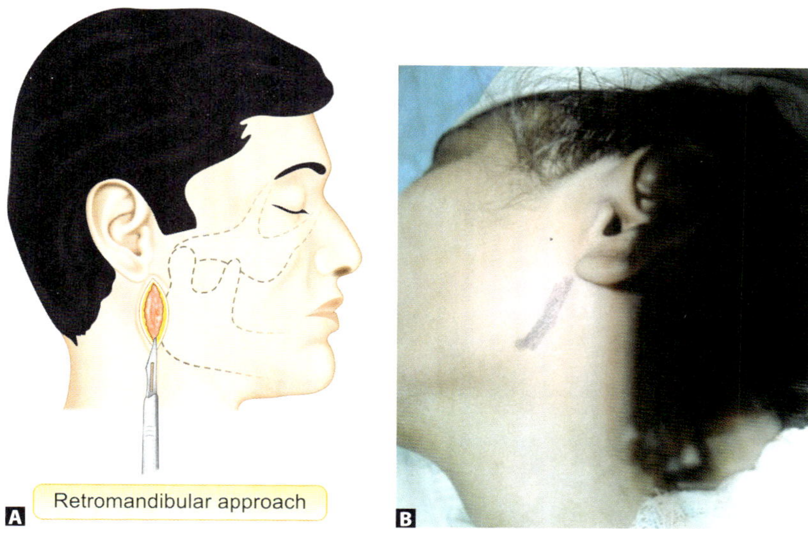

Figs 20A and B: Showing marking for retromandibular incision

Infiltration

Xylocaine 2% + adrenaline (1:200,000).

Resection

- Resection is carried through skin, subcutaneous and thin platysma (Figs 20C and D)

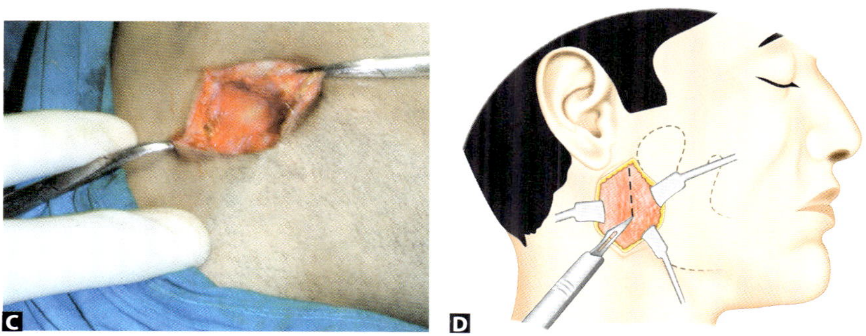

Figs 20C and D: Dissection through skin, subcutaneous and thin platysma

- Superficial musculoaponeurotic system (SMAS) and parotid capsule are incised
- Blunt dissection is carried within the gland in anteromedial direction (Figs 20E and F)

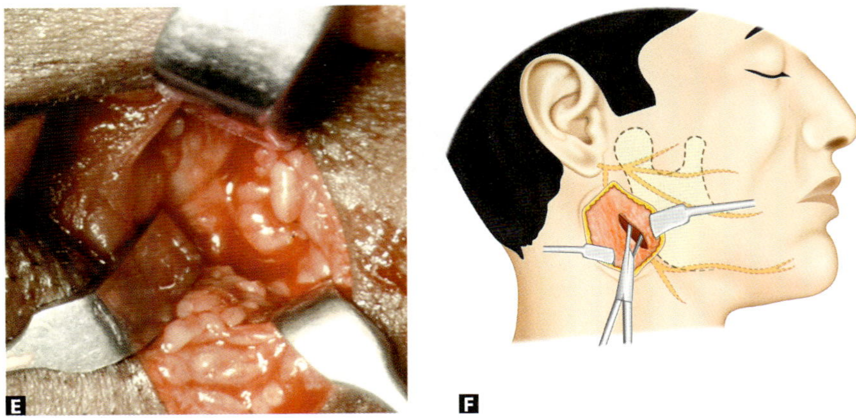

Figs 20E and F: Dissection through parotid in anteromedial direction

- Care must be taken for the identification of external jugular vein
- The marginal mandibulr nerve exits the parotid tail anterior to the external jugular vein (EJV), thus ligating and lifting EJV will secure the nerve (Fig. 20G).

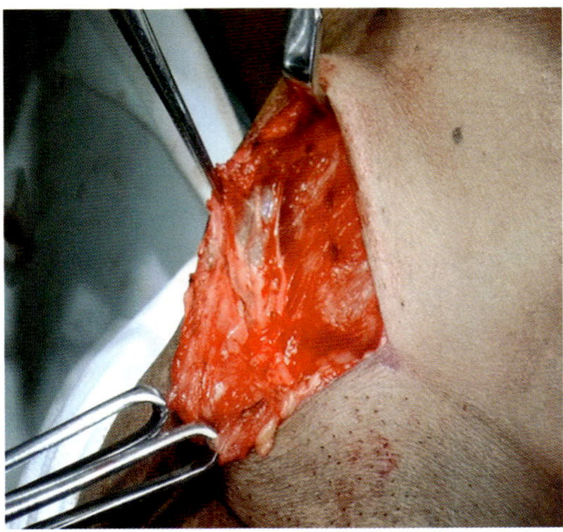

Fig. 20G: Dissection showing EJV and marginal mandibular nerve

- The marginal mandibular nerve and cervical branch of facial nerve are freed from soft tissue and retracted. This will expose pterygomasseteric sling at the posterior border of mandible. This sling is divided with the help of a cautery to expose posterior border of mandible (Figs 20H and I).

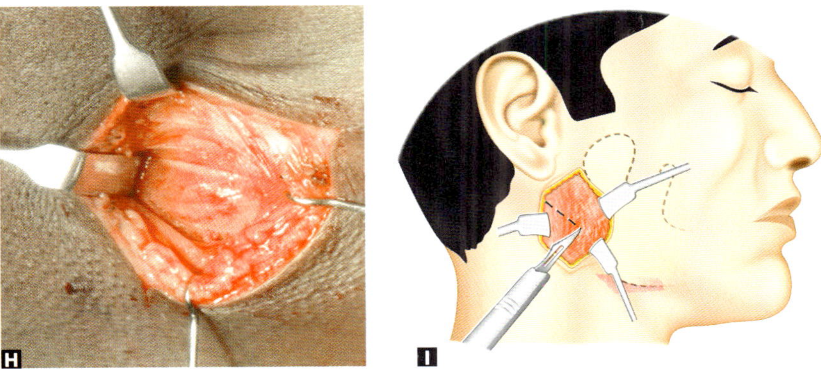

Figs 20H and I: Incision and exposure of pterygomasseteric sling

- Periosteum of the mandible is sharply incised to expose the posterior border of the mandible and the fractured segment is identified and required fixation is done (Fig. 20J).

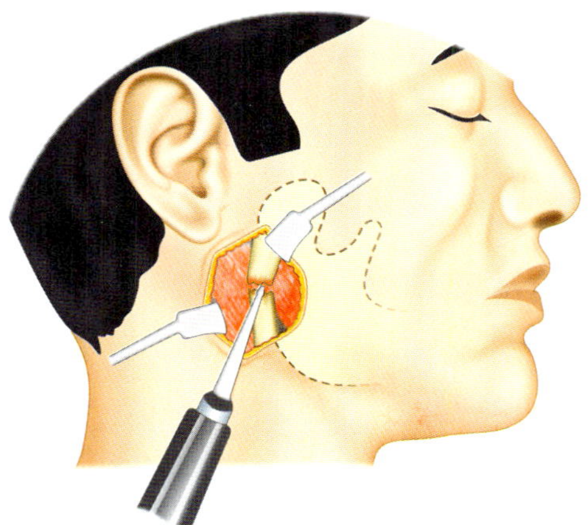

Fig. 20J: Exposure of fracture site

Advantages

- Less conspicuous facial scar
- Good access to posterior border of mandible and sigmoid notch
- It covers shorter distance from incision to condyle.

Disadvantages

- High chances of injuring marginal mandibular nerve
- EJV has to be sacrificed
- Increased chances of salivary fistula and sialocele.

Preauricular Approach

Indications

- It is used for high subcondylar fractures and for access to temporomandibular joint
- Preauricular approach is preferred and is the only option left in cases of anteromedial dislocation or complete medial dislocation of the condylar segment
- For patients reporting very late for surgery with resultant scarring of tissue, preauricular approach is the only option.

Advantages

- It gives direct surgical access to upper condyle and joint space
- It provides excellent access to TMJ during surgical procedures.

Incision

A preauricular incision, 5-6 cm long is made along the curvature of pinna is made. Superiorly, a small temporal extension is made in a foreward arch at about 45° to the zygomatic arch (Figs 21A and B).

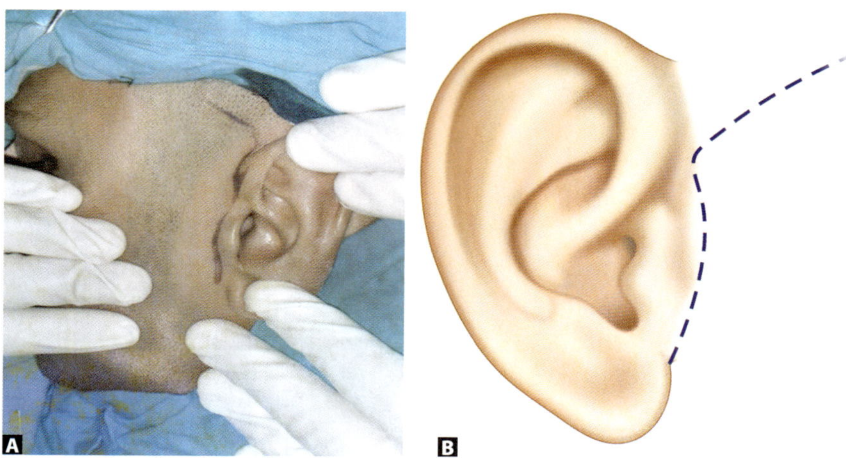

Figs 21A and B: Marking for preauricular incision

Infiltration

Xylocaine 2% + adrenaline (1:200,000)

Dissection

- Skin flap elavated (Fig. 21C).
- Inferiorly, the flap is elevated in avascular plane which is parellel to external auditary canal. This is further elevated anteromedially

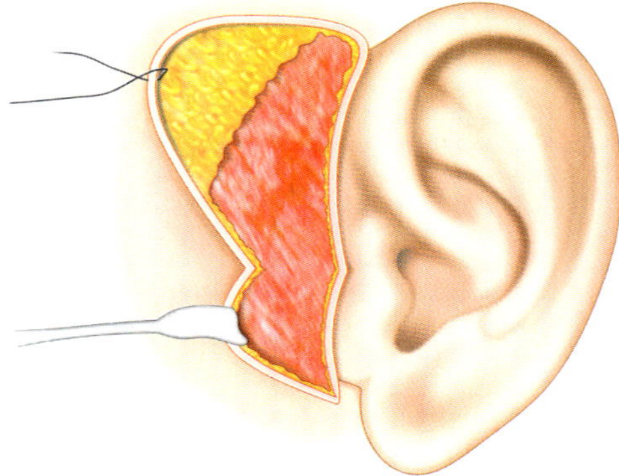

Fig. 21C: Elevation of skin flap

- Superiorly, the flap is elevated till the temporalis fascia is seen (Fig. 21D). Care must be taken to prevent injury to the superficial temporal vessels.

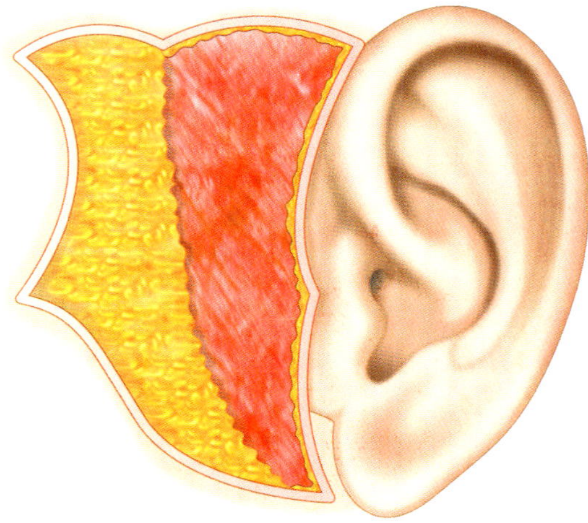

Fig. 21D: Exposure of temporalis fascia

- Once the temporalis fascia is exposed, it is incised in vertical oblique direction parallel to frontal branch of facial nerve above the zygomatic arch (Fig. 21E).

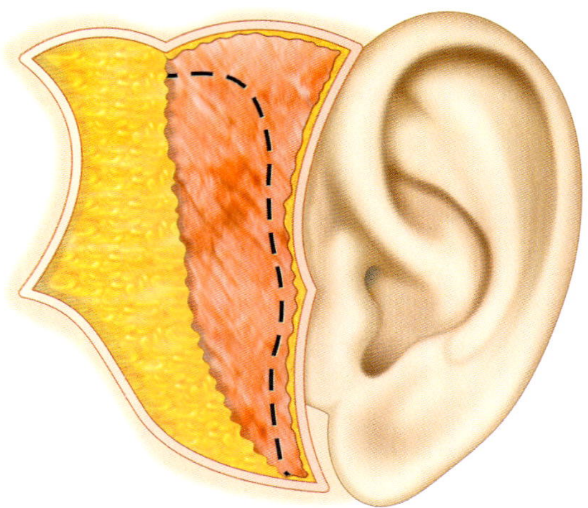

Fig. 21E: Incision is marked in vertical oblique direction parallel to frontal branch of facial nerve above the zygomatic arch

- The frontal branch of facial nerve lies at a distance of 0.8–3.5 cm from postglenoid tubercle. Thus, the incision which is taken over the fascia temporalis, should lie within a distance of 0.8 cm (Fig. 21F).

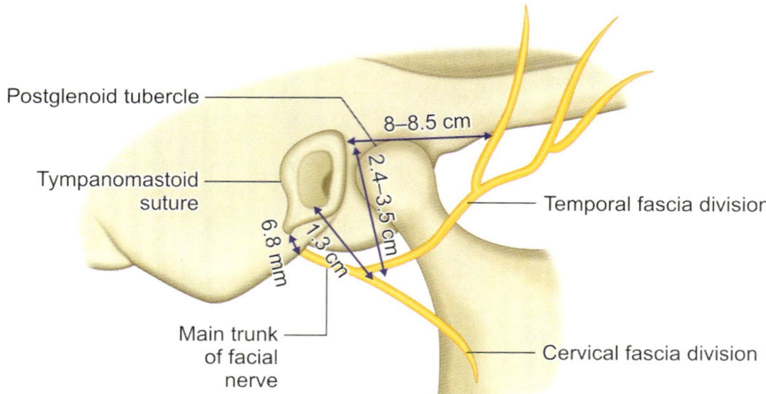

Fig. 21F: Showing distance between frontal branch of facial nerve and postglenoid tubercle

- This incision on the temporalis fascia will retract the frontal branch of facial nerve with the flap. Further dissection is carried out by blunt dissection with periosteum elevator exposing the zygomatic arch

- The assistant is asked to manipulate the mandible so that position of moving condyle can be checked
- Further dissection is carried out to identify the condyle.
- Necessary intervention in the condyle and/or joint is done.

Wound Closure

Wound is closed in the following fashion (Fig. 21G):
- Temoralis fascia layer
- Skin and subcut layer.

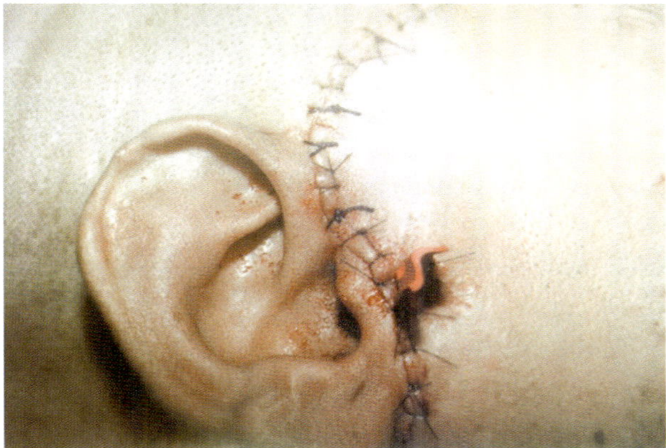

Fig. 21G: Closure of wound in layers

Alterations in Preauricular Incision

1. Facelift Incision

This incision is only taken in preauricular skin crease and extended posteriorly in hairline (Fig. 22A).

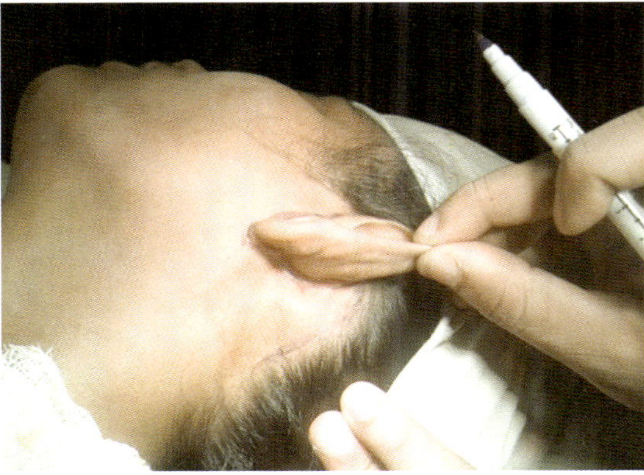

Fig. 22A: Facelift incision

2. Rowe Modification

This is a preauricular incision with temporal extension. The upper part of incision is angled at 45° to the zygomatic arch from the point of attachment of helix.

This incision allows extensive elevation of flap avoiding traction to the upper part of the facial nerve.

3. Blair and Ivy Modification

This is preauricular incision with inverted hockey stick incision over zygomatic arch. This gives easy access and better exposure of zygomatic and condylar arch (Fig. 22B).

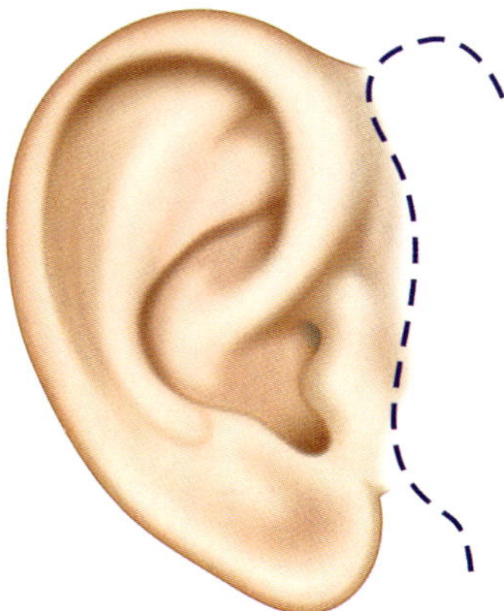

Fig. 22B: Blair's inverted hockey incision

4. Endaural Approach(Lempert and Shambaugh Modification)

Here, the incision is taken over inner aspect of the tragus avoiding direct incision over the face. This gives good scar but the access is limited (Fig. 22C).

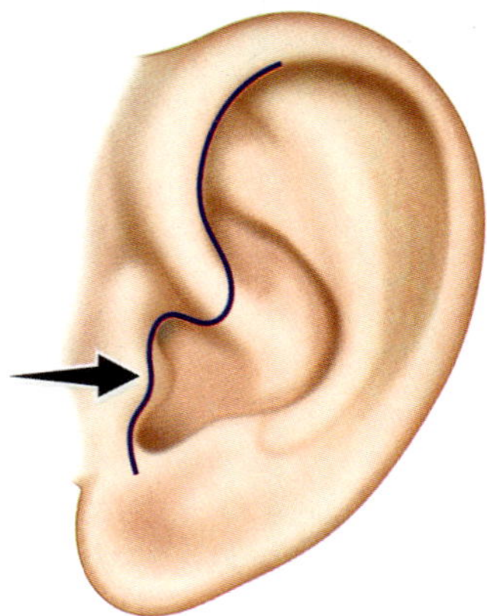

Fig. 22C: Modified endaural incision

5. Alkayat-Bramley Incision

It is a modification of preauricular incision where the upper part of the incision is extended in a question mark fashion over the temporal area to gain better access (Fig. 22D).

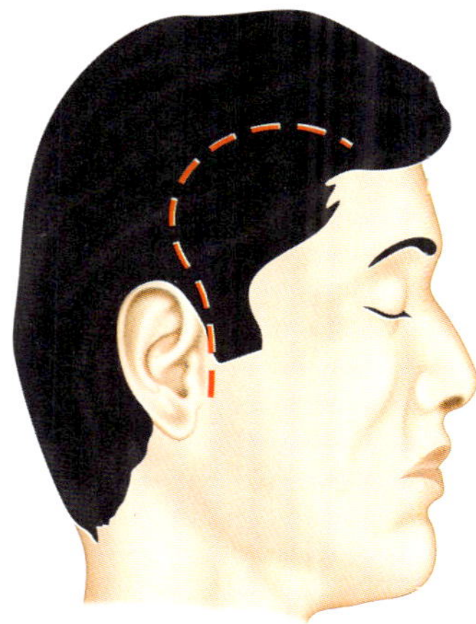

Fig. 22D: Alkayat-Bramley incision

Intraoral Approaches

- The vestibular incision can be used for standard fracture fixation techniques or in conjunction with endoscopically assisted surgical techniques
- The ramus and condylar region can be exposed via an intraoral approach by extending the standard vestibular incision in a superior direction up to the ascending ramus. The incision can be altered depending on the area of the ramus/condylar process that needs exposure and treatment
- Oral contamination is not a contraindication for intraoral incision
- In complex fractures including comminuted and avulsive fractures that require the placement of load-bearing reconstruction plates, a transfacial/extraoral approach can provide better access to treat the injury.

Incision

Unless contraindicated, infiltrate the area with a local anesthetic containing a vasoconstrictor.

Make an incision through the mucosa in the vestibule approximately 5 mm away from the attached gingiva (mucogingival junction), extending up the external oblique ridge (Fig. 23).

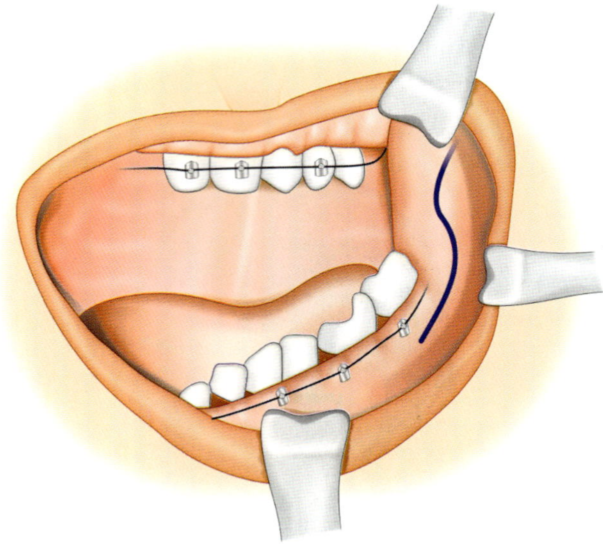

Fig. 23: Incision 5 mm away from the attached gingiva

Exposure of Fracture

The lateral surface of the ramus and condylar process is exposed in a subperiosteal plane to visualize the fracture. Right-angled retractors and fiberoptic lighting would facilitate this procedure. The fracture must be reduced adequately before fixation is applied. The fixation can be done either by transbuccal or right-angled instrumentation.

Endoscopic Approaches

- The surgeon has the option of treating the fracture through the intraoral approach under direct vision or may opt for endoscopic assistance
- A specific instrumentation is recommended in order to facilitate the endoscopically assisted condylar fracture treatment
- Create the optical cavity for the endoscope by elevating the periosteum of the ascending ramus towards the condylar region. Stop the dissection once you have reached the fracture line. Dissection beyond the fracture line will be completed after introduction of the endoscope.

Insertion of the Optical Retractor

After assembling the optical retractor to its handle, insert and place it around the posterior border of the ramus.

Insertion of the Endoscope

Insert the endoscope through the optical retractor up to the fracture line.

Dissect Over the Condylar Fragment

- Using the periosteal elevator dissect under endoscopic visualization over the condylar fragment. Care should be taken near the inferior border of the capsule, not to violate the joint space
- If the condylar fracture fragment is initially medially displaced, the surgeon must bring the fragment into a lateral position in order to complete the dissection for the osteosynthesis
- This may be a highly demanding procedure.

Wound Closure

- Closure of the intraoral incision after thoroughly irrigating the wound and checking for hemostasis
- The incision is closed using interrupted or running resorbable sutures.

Surgical Dressing

An elastic pressure dressing covering the ramus/condylar process region helps support the soft tissues and prevent hematoma formation.

CHAPTER

Approaches to Zygomatic Fracture

APPROACHES TO ZYGOMA

Zygomatic bone is a strong buttress of middle third of facial skeleton in its lateral aspect. There are five articulations in zygoma which get disrupted during trauma.

1. Zygoma articulates with frontal bone forming zygomaticofrontal suture.
2. Zygoma articulates with maxillary bone forming zygomaticomaxillary buttress.
3. It articulates with orbit through inferior orbital rim.
4. It articulates with temporal bone by zygomatic arch.
5. It articulates with sphenoid by zygomaticosphenoid suture.

Zygoma fracture is also called tripod fracture or trimalar fracture (Fig. 1), because there is fracture at three articulated points:

1. Zygomaticofrontal suture
2. Zygomaticomaxillary buttress
3. Inferior orbital rim

Hence, the name called trimalar or tripod fracture.

Treatment

1. Observation
2. Surgery
   a. Close reduction without fixation
   b. Open reduction with fixation.

Four important which things need to be assessed, which decides the management plan of zygoma fractures are:

1. Cosmetic defect or functional deformity—require surgical intervention otherwise it can be well-managed conservatively
2. Isolated or multiple fracture—isolated fracture can be treated by closed reduction while multiple fractures need fixation

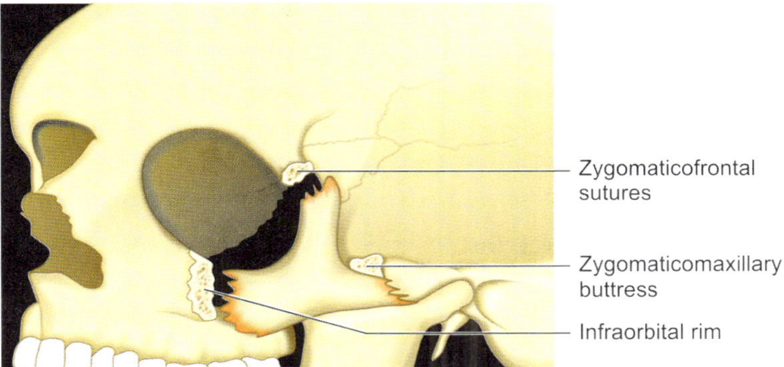

Fig. 1: Tripod fracture

3. Zygomatic arch fracture (medially displaced or laterally displaced):
   - Medially displaced fractures can be treated by closed reduction
   - Laterally displaced needs fixation
4. Complete or incomplete fractures—incomplete fractures need closed reduction, complete fractures need fixation.

Indications of Surgical Management of Zygoma Fractures

- Cosmetic deformity—if there is obvious cosmetic deformity and patient wish to get operated, fracture needs to be addressed.
- Functional disability—to remove any interference with the range of movement of the mandible.
  - Relieve pressure on the infraorbital nerve
  - To correct diplopia
  - For correction of enophthalmos

Surgical Approaches (Flow chart 1)

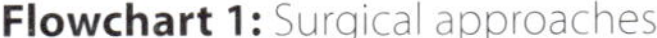

Flowchart 1: Surgical approaches

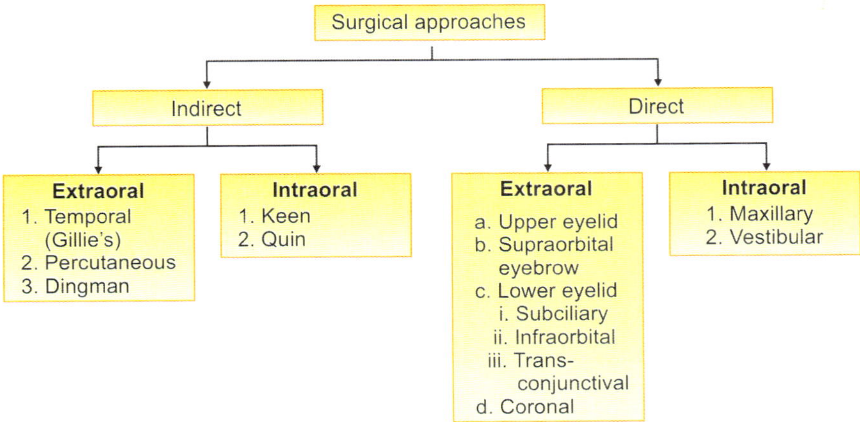

OTHER WAYS OF CLASSIFYING THE APPROACHES

Closed reduction

1. Extraoral
   A. Gillies
   B. Dingman
   C. Percutaneous (towel clip)
2. Intraoral
   A. Keen
   B. Quin

Open reduction

1. Anterior approaches
   A. Zygomaticomaxillary (ZM) buttress
      - Maxillary vestibular incision
        a. Gingivobuccal incision
        b. Sulcular incision
   B. Infraorbital rim
      - Skin incision
        a. Subciliary incision
        b. Midtarsal incision
        c. Infraorbital rim incision
      - Conjunctival incision
   C. Zygomaticofrontal (ZF) suture
        a. Brow incision
        b. Upper lid blepharoplasty
2. Posterior approaches
3. Combined approaches

Closed Reduction

Gillies Temporal Approach

Indications

This approach is used for closed reduction of medially displaced zygomatic arch fractures.

Anatomic Considerations

Temporalis muscle passes beneath the zygomatic arch while the temporalis fascia is attached to the upper border of zygomatic arch (Fig. 2).

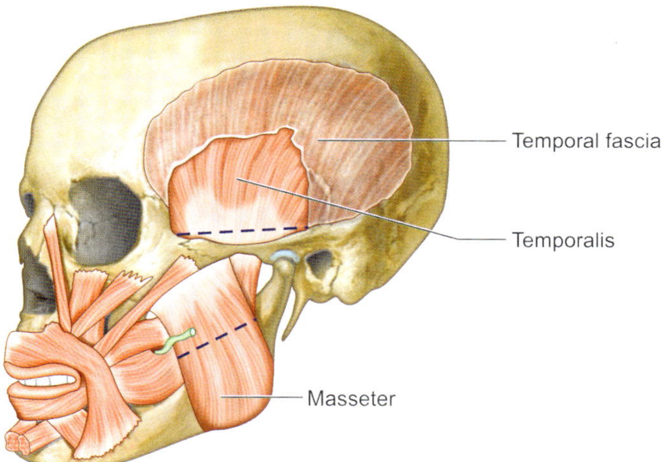

Fig. 2: Temporalis muscle passing beneath the zygomatic arch

Beneath the fascia and above the muscle there lies a potential space wherein an instrument can be passed and engaged to this impacted medially displaced fracture. This forms the principle of Gillies temporal approach (Fig. 3).

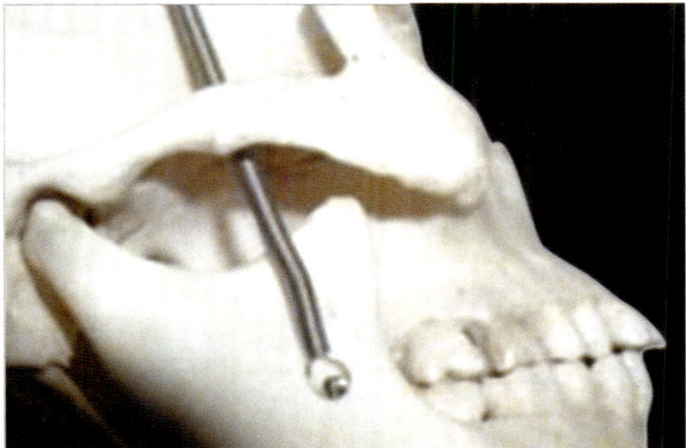

Fig. 3: Depicting the potential space forming the principle of Gillies approach

Steps

1. *Anesthesia*: The procedure is done under general anesthesia.

2. *Position of patient*: Head is turned to opposite side and fracture site is adequately exposed.
3. *Marking*: The zygoma and medially displaced fracture is marked with a marking pen so that the site of fracture is properly determined (Fig. 4A).

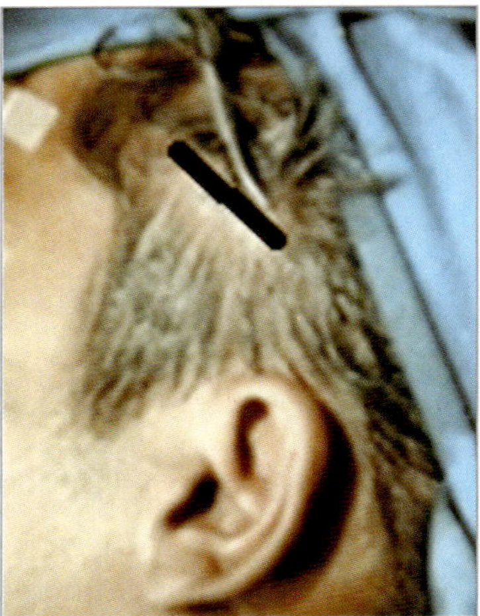

Fig. 4A: Marking of the incision

4. *Incision*: A 2.5 cm horizontal incision at an angle of 45° to the upper border of external ear is placed after 2% lignocaine with adrenaline infiltration. Utmost care is taken not to injure the superficial temporal artery (Fig. 4B).

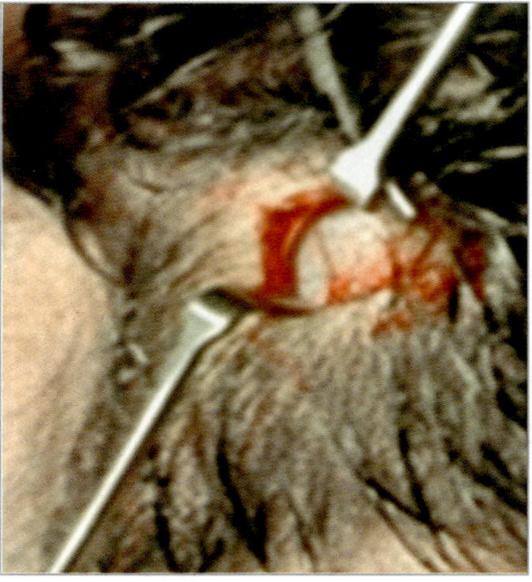

Fig. 4B: Making of incision

5. *Dissection*: Further dissection is carried out till temporalis fascia is identified and incision is taken on temporalis fascia (Fig. 4C).

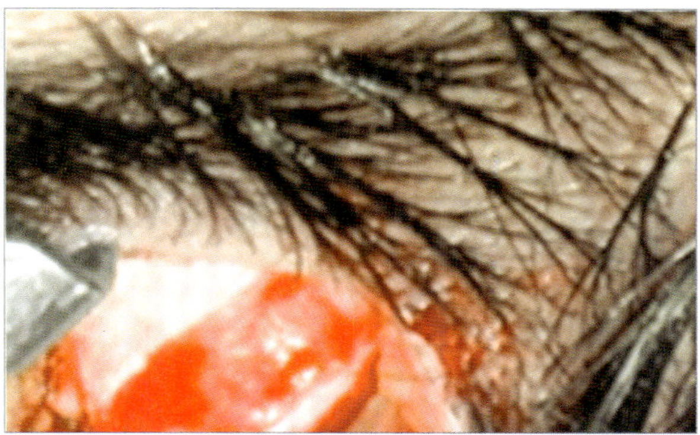

Fig. 4C: Temporalis fascia exposed and cut

6. Rowe's elevator is passed beneath the fascia till it reaches below the zygomatic arch (Figs 4D and E).

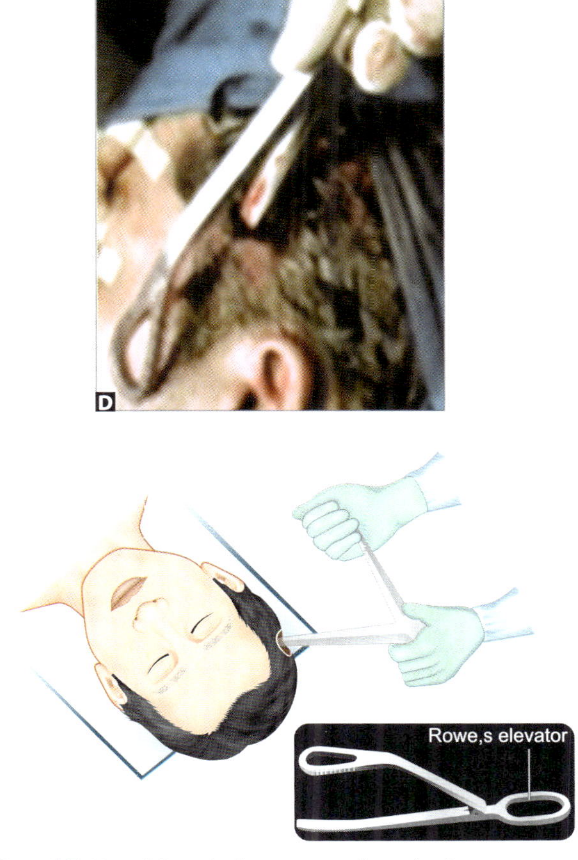

Figs 4D and E: Use of Rowe's elevator to reduce the fracture segment

7. The other arm of the Rowe's elevator will guide about the the arm which is inserted inside.
8. A Bestow elevator (Fig. 4F) can be used alternatively for reduction of the fracture.
9. *Reduction*: With continuous palpation, slowly the arch is reduced by pushing the arch laterally. Care must be taken not to exert too much force on temporal skull as a fulcrum.
10. *Wound closure*: Incision is closed in layers.
11. *Postoperative care*: Patient is asked not to sleep on the fracture side for 7–10 days as this may displace the fracture back.

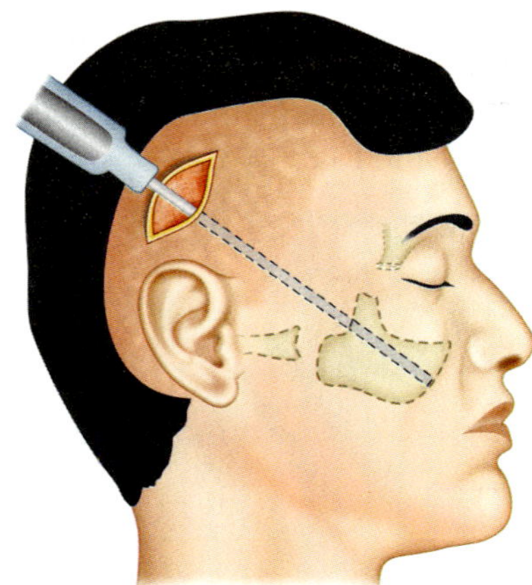

Fig. 4F: Bestow elevator used for elevating medially displaced zygoma arch

Dingman's Approach

In 1964, Dingman and Native described this approach. This is a supraorbital approach which is used for reducing medially displaced zygomatic arch and body.

Steps

1. *Anesthesia*: The procedure is done under general anesthesia.
2. *Position of patient*: Head is turned to opposite side and fracture site is adequately exposed.
3. *Marking*: The zygoma and medially displaced fracture is marked with a marking pen so that the site of fracture is properly determined.
4. *Incision*: Incision is taken adjacent to ipsilateral eyebrow which is near to zygomaticofrontal suture line.

5. *Dissection*: Dissection is carried out till temporalis aponeurosis is identified and the elevator is passed below it. This elevator is passed below the zygomatic arch and body of zygoma and is lifted forward and laterally (Fig. 5).
6. *Closure*: Wound is closed in layers.
7. *Postoperative care*: Patient is asked not to sleep on the side of fracture side for 7–10 days as this may displace the fracture back.

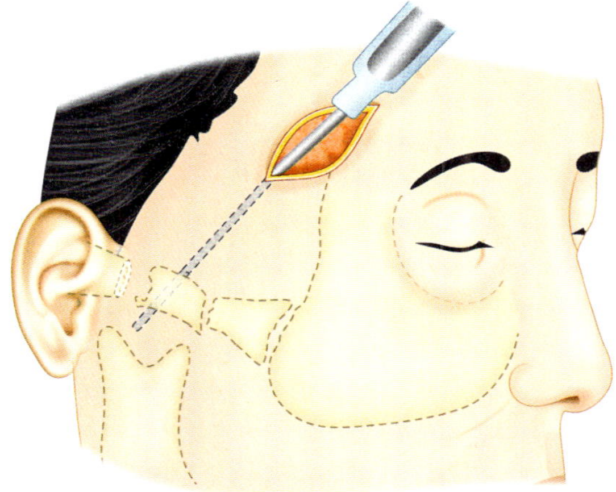

Fig. 5: Supraorbital approach used for the reduction of zygoma bone fracture

Percutaneous Approach

It is also called *towel clip reduction* technique.

Advantages

- Simple technique
- No heavier instruments are required.

Disadvantages

We need to wait till the edema settles and medially displaced segment is distinctly visualized.

Indications

Closed reduction for medially displaced fractures.

Steps

1. Usually done in general anesthesia
2. Position—supine position with face turned to opposite side
3. Marking—zygoma arch is precisely marked including medially displaced fragment (Fig. 6A).

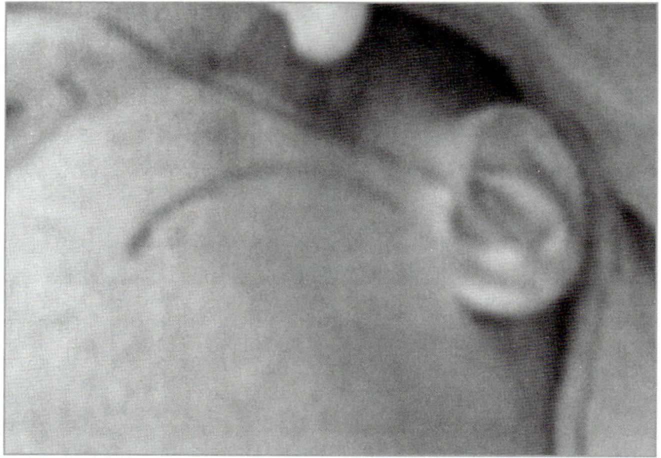

Fig. 6A: Marking of zygoma arch

4. Incision—at upper border of zygoma, at the site of medially displaced fracture (Fig. 6B)

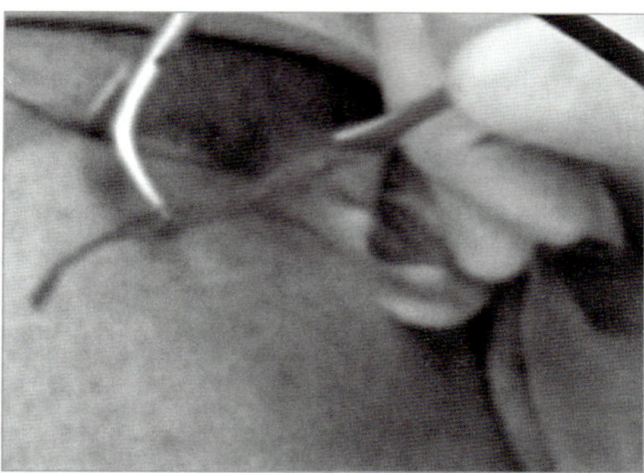

Fig. 6B: Making of incision

5. One end of towel hook is inserted below the zygoma (Fig. 6C)

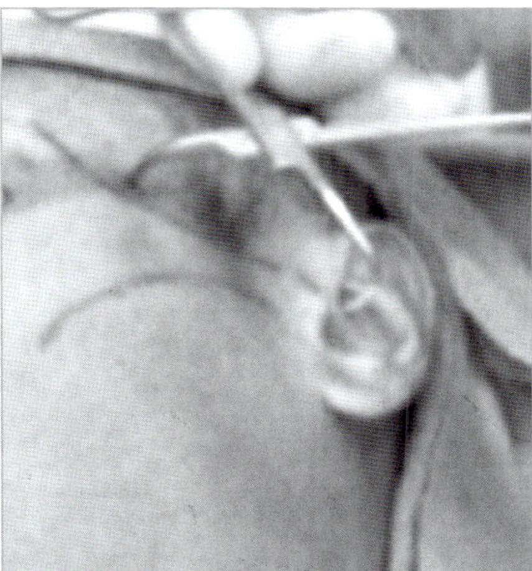

Fig. 6C: Inserting one end of the hook

6. Now the second incision is taken at the lower border of zygoma at the same site of displaced fracture. The second end of towel hook is inserted below the fracture fragment

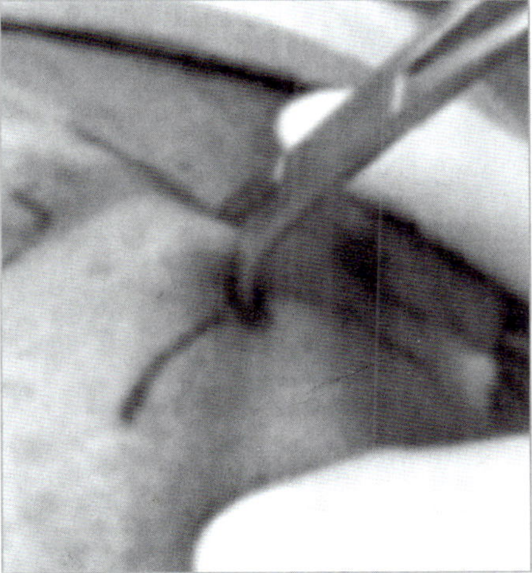

Fig. 6D: Hook is used for the reduction of zygoma fracture

7. Gradually the fracture fragment is reduced (Fig. 6D)
8. Incision is either sutured with 5-0 silk or left alone.

Keen Technique

- It is an intraoral approach also known as buccal sulcus approach
- Keen published an article on this technique in 1909.

Advantages

- It is an intraoral approach
- No external scar is given.

Disadvantages

- There are chances of prolapse of buccal fat
- Care must be taken not to enter into orbit.

Indications

Medially displaced zygomatic arch fractures.

Steps

1. *Anesthesia*: Usually done in general anesthesia.
2. *Position*: Supine with head in neutral position.
3. *Infiltration*: Two percent lignocaine with adrenaline is injected into mucobuccal fold on the side of zygoma fracture.
4. *Marking*: Zygoma arch is precisely marked including medially displaced fragment.
5. *Incision*: A 1 cm incision is made in the mucobuccal fold, just beneath the zygomatic buttress of the maxilla (Fig. 7A).

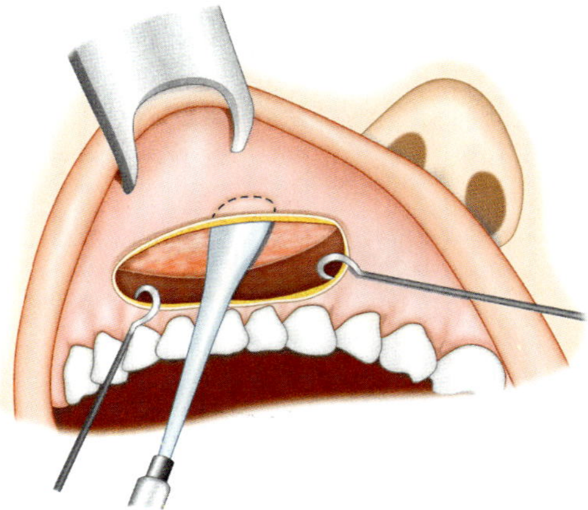

Fig. 7A: Incision made in mucobuccal fold

6. *Dissection and elevation*: A heavier instrument can then be inserted behind the infratemporal surface of the zygoma. Superior, lateral, and anterior force is applied with the instrument to reduce the bone (Fig. 7B).

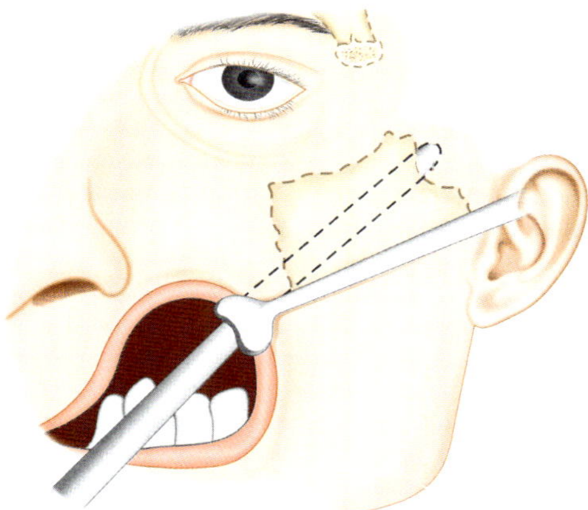

Fig. 7B: A heavier instrument is used for the reduction of zygoma bone

7. *Closure*: Wound is closed in layers.

Carroll-Girard Approach

This is a transcutaneous cheek approach.

Advantages

- Screw available provides flexible manipulation and ability to position the zygoma
- The technique is flexible, especially useful in laterally displaced fracture
- Useful in fracture which is several days old and the masseter is slightly contracted
- Used as a closed approach or during open reduction
- Can be used for medially displaced fractures.

Disadvantages

Special instruments are required for this technique.

Steps

1. *Anesthesia*: General anesthesia is required
2. *Position*: Position with face turned to opposite side
3. *Infiltration*: Two percent lignocaine with adrenaline is injected over the inferior tubercle of malar prominence.

4. *Incision*: A 3 mm incision is taken directly over the inferior tubercle of malar prominence
5. *Dissection*: Dissection is carried out with a clamp which is spread along the direction of facial nerve until the periosteum of zygomatic body is encountered
6. A small hole of appropriate size is drilled in bone (Fig. 8)
7. Bone screw is inserted in the hole
8. Precaution must be taken during making a hole that adjacent soft tissue is not damaged

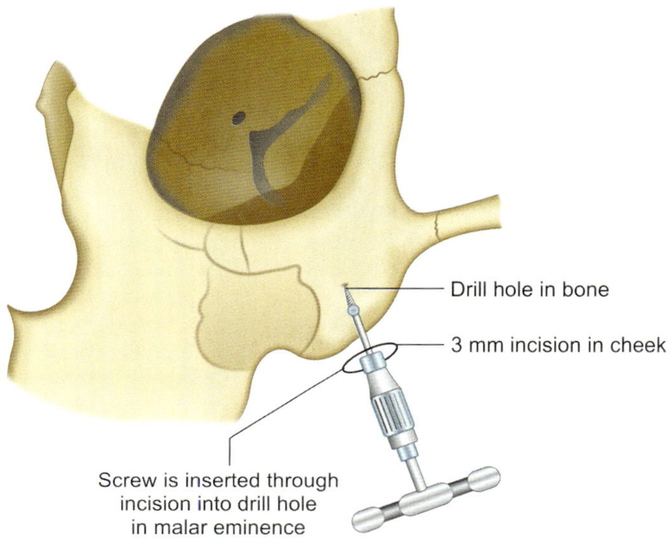

Fig. 8: Girard screw is used for the reduction of fracture

9. Adequate manipulation is done and the fracture segment is reduced (Fig. 8)
10. Wound is closed or left alone.

OPEN REDUCTION

1. Anterior approaches (Fig. 9)
   A. Infraorbital rim
   B. Zygomaticofrontal suture
   C. Zygomaticomaxillary buttress

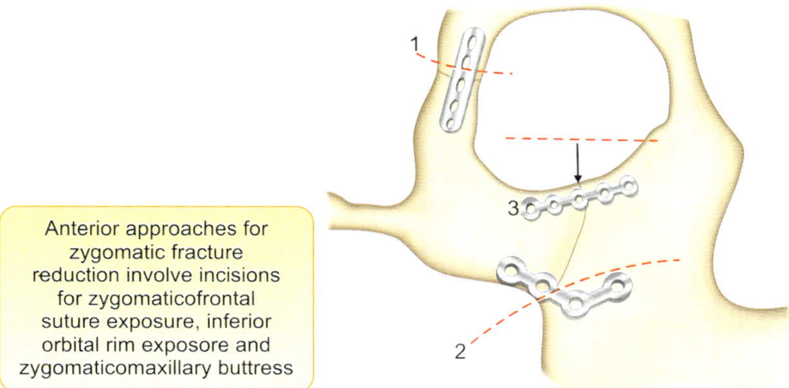

Fig. 9: Anterior approaches for (1) zygomaticofrontal suture line, (2) zygomaticomaxillary buttress and (3) infraorbita rim

2. Posterior approaches (Fig. 10)
   A. Lateral orbital wall
   B. Zygomatic arch

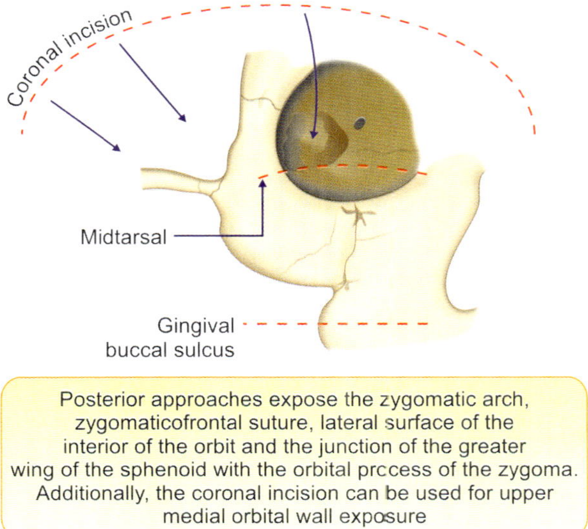

Fig. 10: Posterior approaches used for zygomatic arch and lateral orbital wall

3. Combined approach (anterior + posterior).

ANTERIOR APPROACHES

Zygomaticomaxillary Buttress

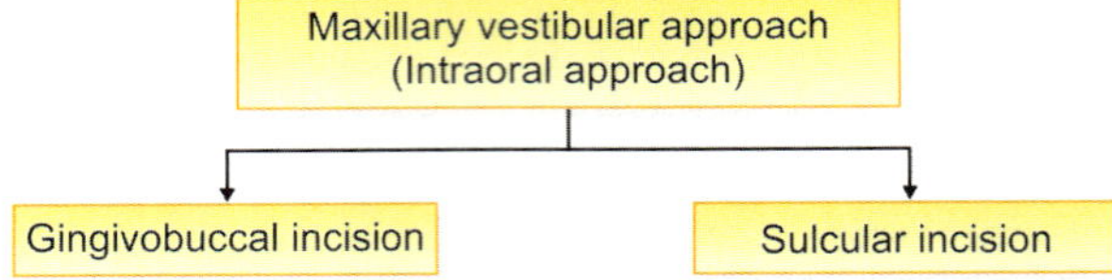

Gingivobuccal Incision

This is a typical incision which we use for Caldwell Luc procedures.

Advantages

- No external scar is seen
- It is an intraoral approach.

Disadvantage

- Chances of wound dehiscence.

Steps

1. Incision is taken over mucosa 4 to 5 mm beyond the level of attached gingiva (Fig. 11).

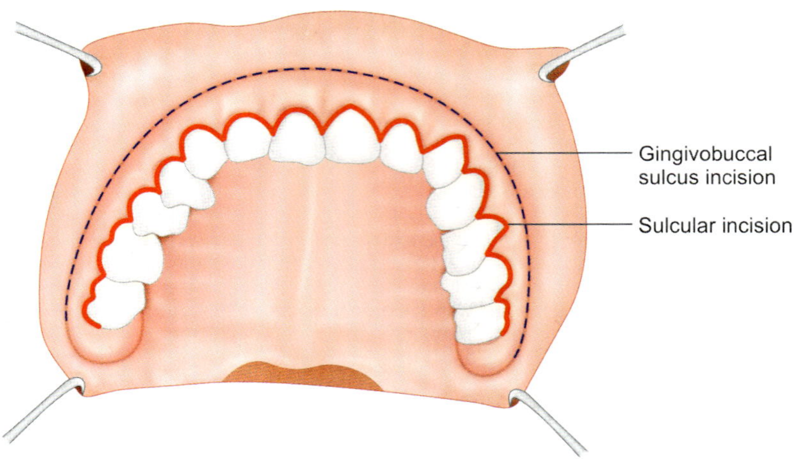

Fig. 11: Dotted line shows gingivobuccal sulcus incision while dark continuous incision mark show sulcular incision

2. Infiltration is done at the incision site
3. Dissection is carried out till the periosteum of maxilla is seen, fracture site is exposed, reduced and fixed
4. Wound is closed in layers.

Marginal Gingival Incision (Sulcular Incision)

Advantages

- Minimal scar formation
- Less chances of infection
- Wound dehiscence is never seen with this approach.

Steps

1. Incision is taken along the gingiva attached to teeth (Fig. 11)
2. Dissection is similar as earlier
3. Wound is closed in layers. Suture is passed through teeth as intermaxillary fixation.

Infraorbital Rim Approach

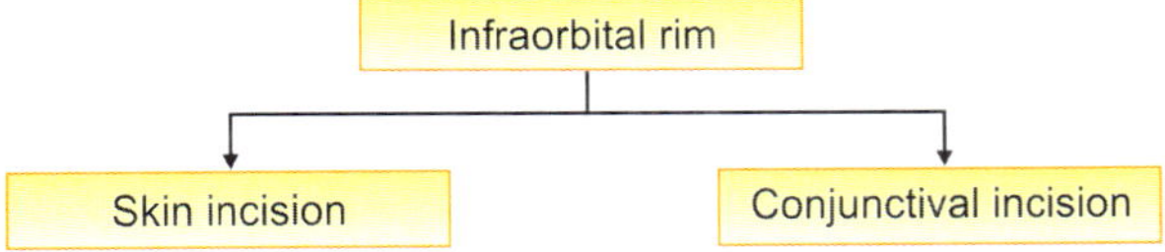

Skin Incision

1. Subciliary incision
   a. Standard incision
   b. Converse subciliary incision
2. Midtarsal incision
3. Infraorbital rim incision.

Anatomic Considerations

The different layers of lower eyelid are (Fig. 12):

- Skin
- Subcutaneous tissue
- Orbicularis oculi muscle
- Orbital septum

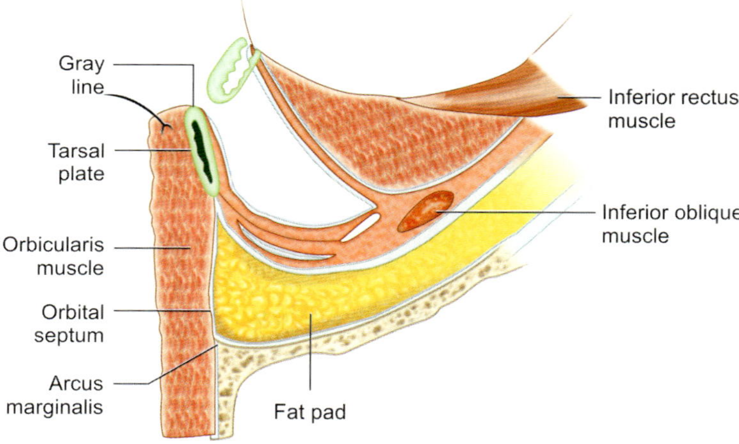

Fig. 12: Various layers of lower eyelid

- Orbital fat
- Inferior oblique muscle.

Important Considerations

Isolated skin flap should not be elevated as it is a random skin flap. Elevation of this skin flap can lead to infarction of skin and there are increased chances of vertical lid shortening leading to scleral show and ectropian.

Always skin muscle flap has to be used as there are less chances of vertical lid shortening and scleral show.

The orbital septa of lower eyelid is a continuation of mucoperiosteum layer of maxilla layer which lies in between orbicularis muscle and orbital fat. Its lower end is attached few millimeters below orbital rim.

All precautions have to be taken to prevent breach in orbital septum to prevent prolapse of orbital fat.

Incision in infraorbital rim periosteum is taken few millimeters below the rim to prevent injury to orbital septa.

Subciliary Incision (See Fig. 18)

1. Standard Incision

Steps

1. Temporary tarsorrhaphy is done to protect the eyeball (Fig. 13).

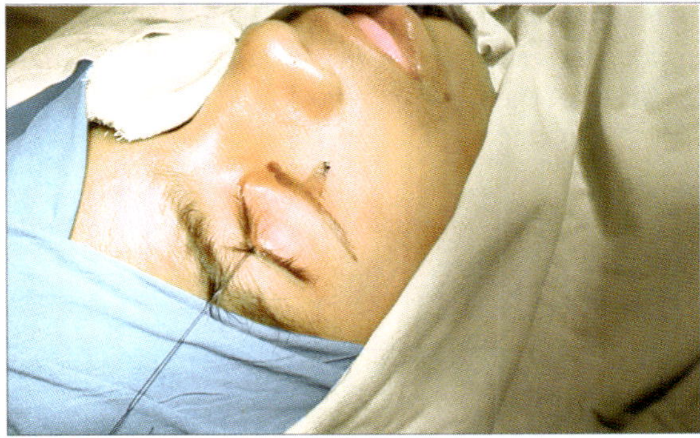

Fig. 13: Temporary tarsorrhaphy

2. Incision is taken 2 to 3 mm below the eyelashes and extended only 8 to 10 mm lateral to lateral canthus (Fig. 14).

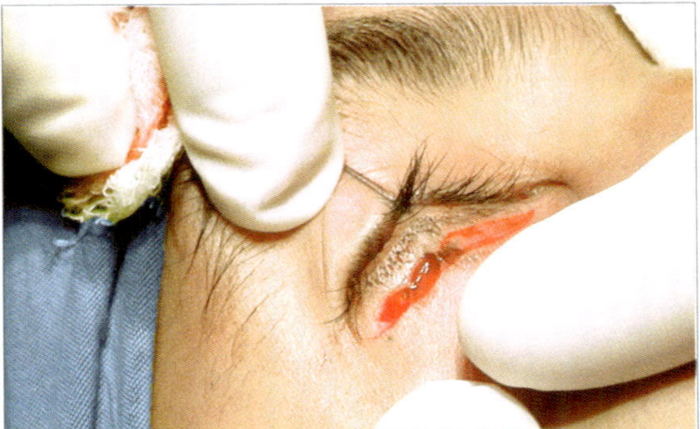

Fig. 14: Incision is taken few mm below the eyelashes

3. Avoid extension of this incision into cheek as this leads to noticeable scar.
4. Skin muscle flap is elevated till the infraorbital rim is reached (Fig. 15).

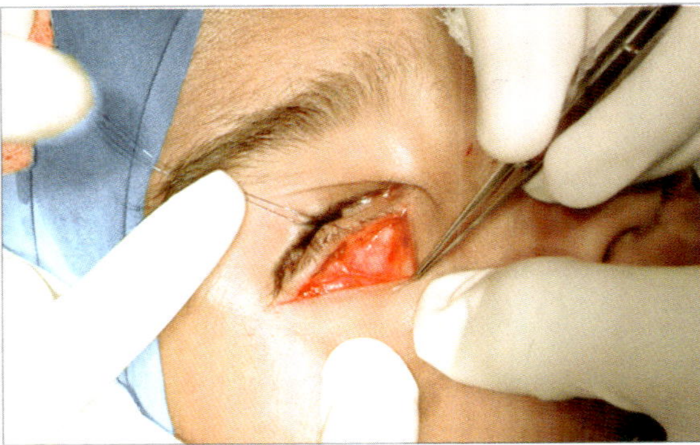

Fig. 15: Exposure of orbital septum

5. Utmost care is taken to prevent injury to orbital septa.
6. At infraorbital rim, periosteum is incised few millimeters below the infraorbital rim to prevent injury to orbital septa, thus infraorbital rim is exposed, reduced and fixed (Figs 16A and B).

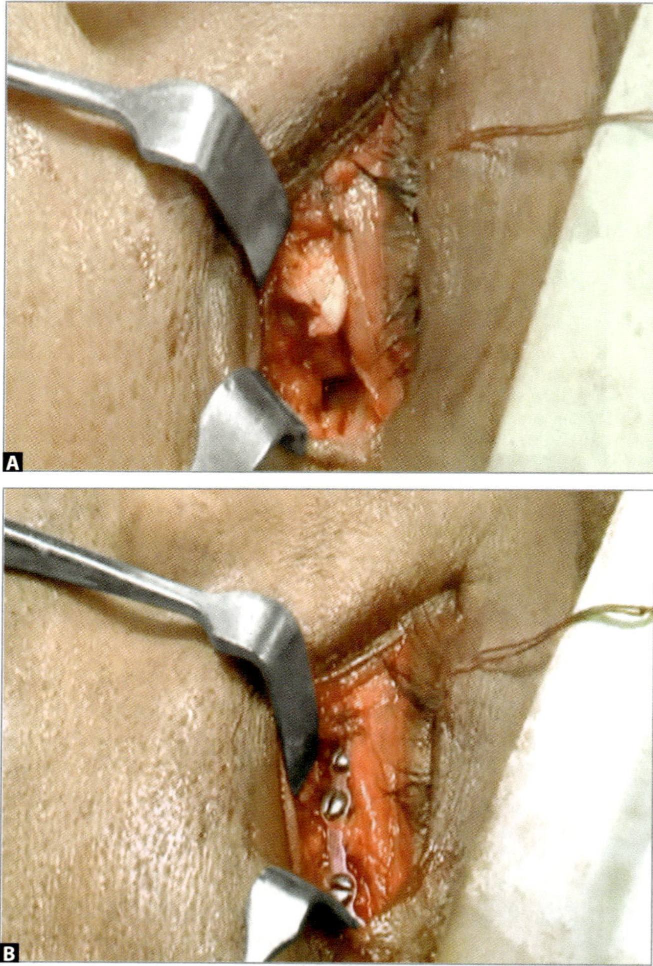

Figs16A and B: Exposure and fixation of implant

7. The periosteal edge of the incision can be marked with fine silk suture and cut short on each side to identify the edge of closure.
8. Wound is then closed in layers (Fig. 17).

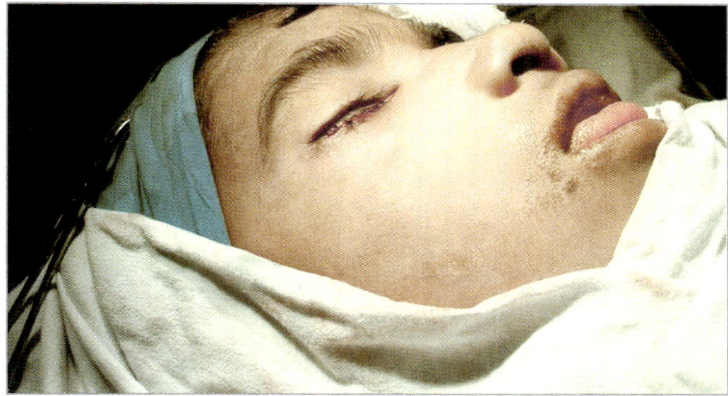

Fig. 17: Wound closure

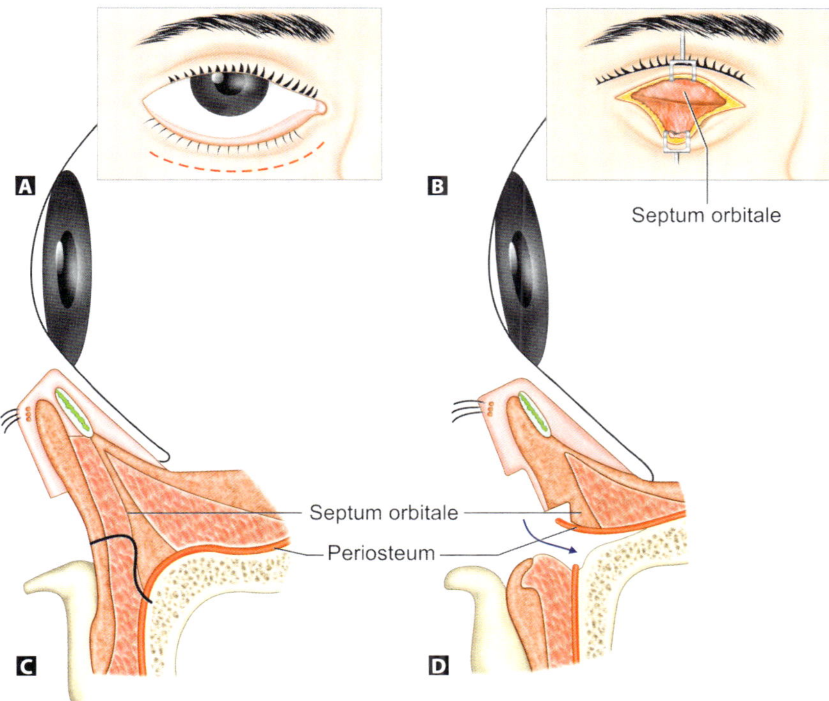

Figs 18A to D: Subciliary incision: (A) Marking of incision few mm below the eyelashes; (B) Elevation of the myocutaneous flap; (C) Incision over the periosteum below the attachment of orbital septum; (D) Exposure of the orbital rim

Disadvantages

- Highest incidence of lid retraction
- Increased chances of scleral show
- Increased chances of ectropion.

2. Converse Subciliary Incision

- The incision is taken 2 to 3 mm below the eyelashes
- Only skin flap is elevated for few millimeters, thus resecting superficial to tarsal orbicularis muscle and preventing injury to the same (Fig. 19)

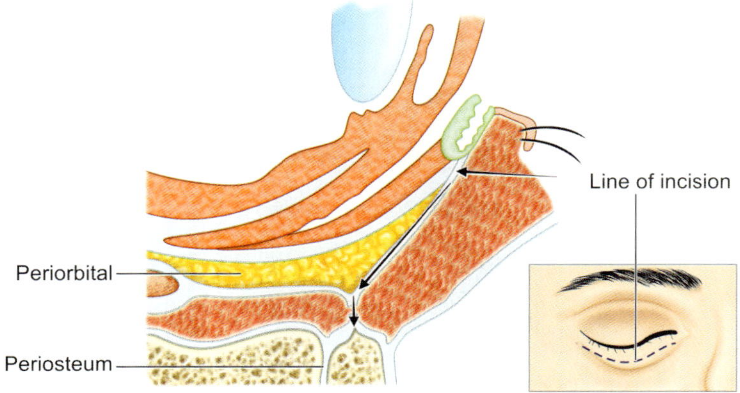

Fig. 19: Showing converse subciliary incision wherein skin flap is elevated for few millimeters and then skin muscle flap is elevated

- Below, the tarsal plate incision is taken over the orbicularis muscle, thus raising the skin muscle flap till infraorbital rim
- This incision prevents injury to orbicularis oculi part of tarsal plate, thus reducing chances of ectropion and lid retraction
- At infraorbital rim the periosteum is incised few millimeters below the infraorbital rim to prevent injury to orbital septa, thus infraorbital rim is exposed, reduced and fixed
- The periosteal edge of the incision can be marked with fine silk suture and cut short on each side to identify the edge of closure.

Midtarsal Incision (Fig. 20)

- Incision is taken at the lower eyelid crease (1 mm below the midtarsal crease in the lid)
- Skin muscle flap is elevated
- Rest of the dissection is similar to subciliary approach.

Advantages

This incision do not denervate the pretarsal orbicularis occuli muscle leading to less chances of ectropion and scleral show.

Disadvantages

Scar is more visible than subciliary incision.

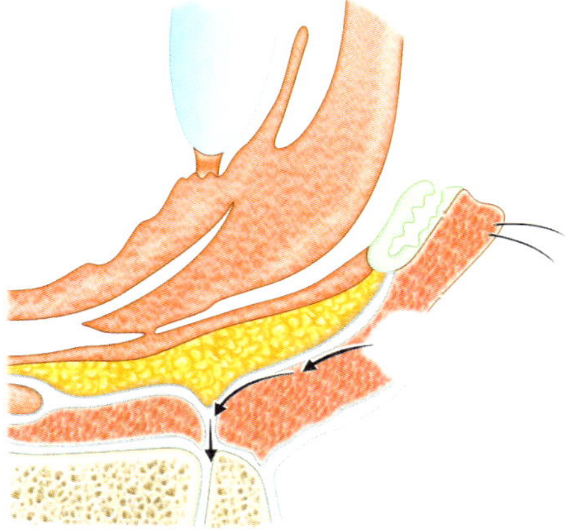

Fig. 20: Midtarsal incision

Infraorbital Rim Incision

Incision is taken directly on infraorbital rim (Fig. 21).

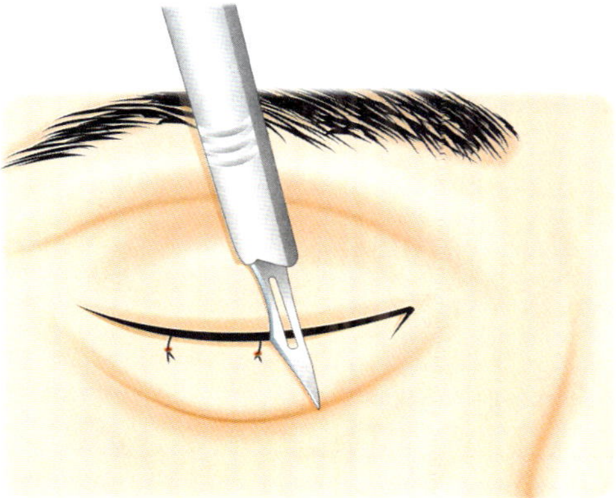

Fig. 21: Infraorbital rim incision

Disadvantage

This incision gives very bad scar.

Conjunctival Incision

- Advocated by Tessir and Converse in 1973
- They used this incision for craniofacial anomalies.

Advantages

- No scar seen
- Lower incidence of ectropion
- Less chances of lid shortening.

Disadvantages

- Restricted access
- Limited extension
- Greater degree of operative dexterity is required, if complications have to be avoided.

Surgical Steps

- Corneal protector is placed over the eye to protect cornea and globe from instrument, retractor or drill
- Traction sutures are taken in lower lid and inferior conjunctival fornices for retraction and eversion of lower lid.

Infiltration and Incision

- Two percent lignocaine with adrenaline is infiltrated. Needle is inserted between the conjunctiva and the tarsal plate, and subsequently inserted again through the skin deep to the palpebral portion of the orbicularis oculi but superficial to septum. Conjunctival incision below the lower border of tarsus is taken on the medial aspect and in line of punctum (Fig.22).

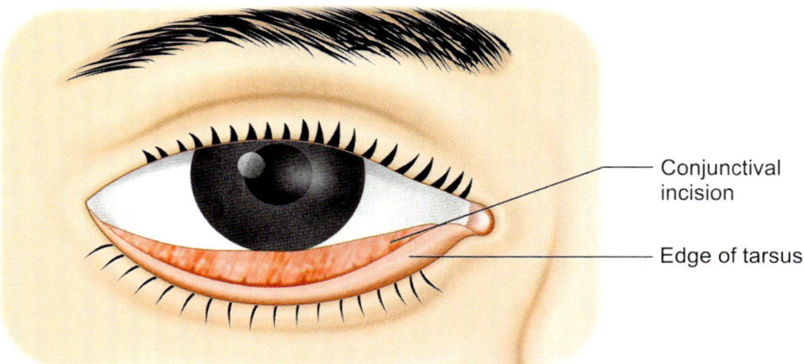

Fig. 22: Conjunctival incision

- For the incision, scissors/scalpels or electrocautery can be used. Lower eyelid retractors are undermined toward the inner angle of the lids. Fat compartment and septum are identified, and dissection is carried out anterior to septum and posterior to orbicularis oculi muscle (Fig. 23).

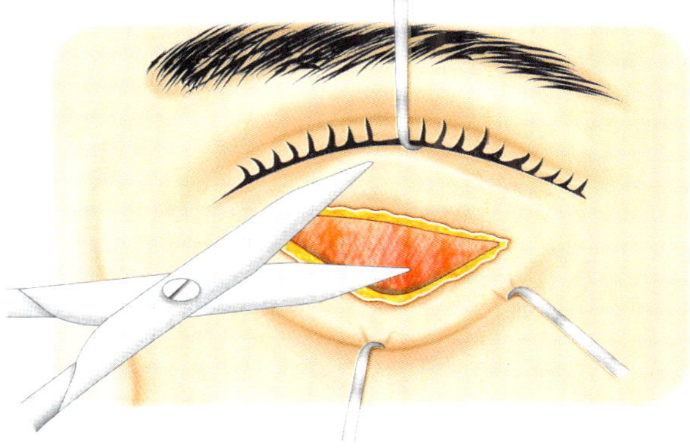

Fig. 23: Flap created just anterior to orbital septum and posterior to orbicularis muscle

- The dissection is carried out till infraorbital rim is reached (Figs 24 and 25). Further steps are same as subciliary incision.

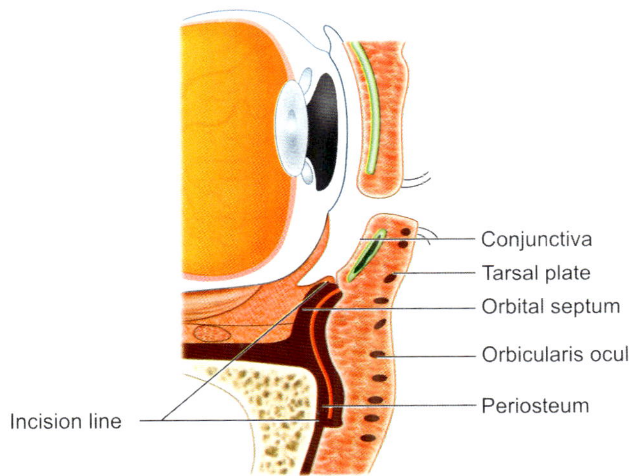

Fig. 24: Schematic diagram for conjunctival incision

Wound Closure

Wound is closed in layers. First the periosteum over the periorbital rim is closed and then conjunctival layers are closed with 6.0 vicryl. The conjunctival flaps must be aligned accurately.

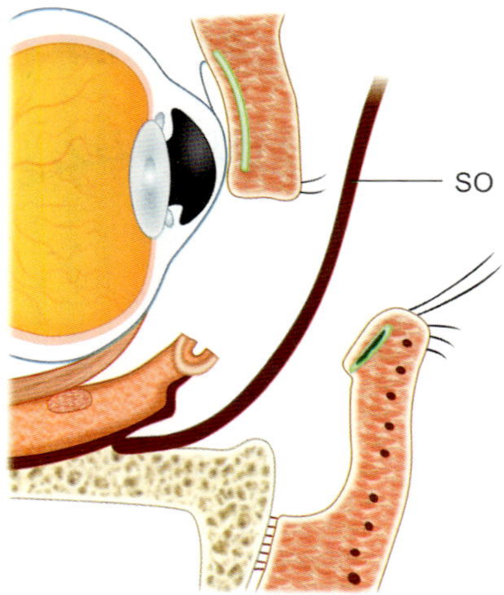

Fig. 25: Dissection carried out to expose the infraorbital rim

Postoperative Positioning

- Keeping the patient's head in an upright position, both preoperatively and postoperatively may significantly improve periorbital edema and pain.
- Avoid nose-blowing to prevent orbital emphysema; nose-blowing should be avoided for at least 10 days following orbital fracture repair.

Wound Care

- Remove sutures from skin after approximately 5 days, if nonresorbable sutures have been used. Apply ice packs (may be effective in a short-term to minimize edema)
- Avoid sun exposure and tanning to skin incisions for several months.

Clinical Follow-up

The patient needs to be examined and reassessed regularly.

Complications

- *Infraorbital paresthesia*: This occurs due to stretching of nerve during retraction. It normally improves in 2–3 weeks
- *Maxillary sinusitis*: These complications may occur due to endoscopic repair
- Eyelid malposition like entropion
- Eye lid laxity

- *Sclera show*: These complications occur due to subciliary approach. These conditions improve in 3–4 weeks
- *Lagophthalmos*: This occurs due to conjunctival approach. It resolves eventually.

Special Instruments

- *Corneal shield*: This is to protect cornea, globe from instrument, retractor or drill
- *Copper malleable retractors of various sizes and shapes*: These are used to retract the orbital globe away from floor without exerting too much pressure on the globe
- *Suitable implant*
- *Fine scissors* for dissection
- *Fine tipped forceps*
- *Glue*
- *1.5 mm × 6 mm screw and 1 mm drill bit to secure implant at anterior orbital rim.*

BICORONAL APPROACH (BITEMPORAL APPROACH)

Following areas are exposed:
- Zygomatic arch
- Lateral orbital rim
- Frontal sinus
- Lateral skull base
- Nasal dorsum
- Temporomandibular joint
- Condylar/subcondylar region
- Ethmoidal sinus
- Entire calvarial vault.

Surgical Consideration

- Scalp consists of 5 layers which can be easily remembered with the mnemonic "SCALP" (Fig. 26).
  - **S**—Skin
  - **C**—Subcutaneous tissue
  - **A**—Aponeurosis and muscles
  - **L**—Loose areolar tissue
  - **P**—Pericranium (Periosteum).

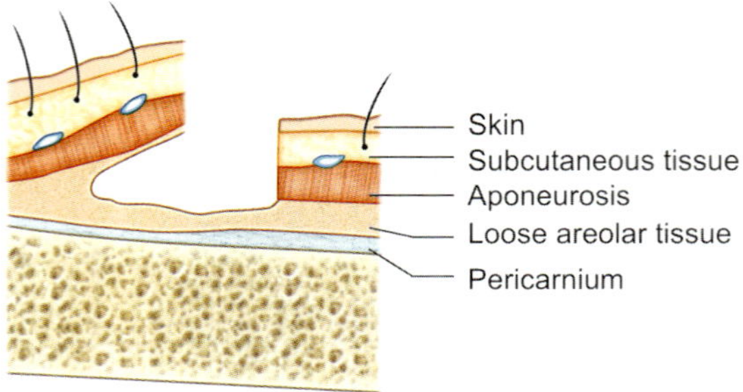

Fig. 26: Various layers of the SCALP

- The skin and subcutaneous tissue in scalp is inseparable.
- The next layer, musculoaponeurotic layer is referred as *Galea*. It cosists of 2 muscles; frontalis and occipital. This galea aponeurosis gives origin to frontalis muscle. Galea is a dense glistering sheet of fibrous tissue which is approximately 0.5 mm, stretching between occipitalis and frontalis muscles. The lateral extension of this aponeurosis in temporoparietal region is known as temporoparietal fascia.
- The loose areolar layer is usually referred as subgaleal plane or subaponeurotic plane. This layer forms a cleavage between galea and periosteum. Anteriorly, subgaleal fascia is continous with loose areolar layer deep to the orbicularis occuli muscle.
- Pericranium is the periostium of the skull. This is firmly attached to the cranial suture lines.

Layers of Temporoparietal Region

This is also called as superficial temporalis fascia or zygomatic SMAS. This fascia is lateral extension of galea and is continuous with SMAS of face.

The superficial temporalis fascia is divided along an oblique line from the level of tragus to supraorbital ridge to enter the temporal fat pad. This division of fascia protects the temporal branch of facial nerve from injury as frontal branch of facial nerve lies superficial to superficial temporal fascia.

Incision

Incision line depends upon:
- Hairline of the patient
- Area to be accessed.

Hair Line

- Incision is taken few millimeters posterior to the hair line (Fig. 27A).

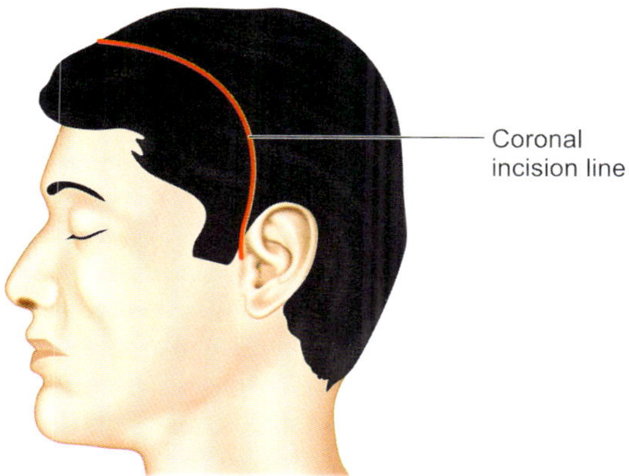

Fig. 27A: Coronal incision in normal hair bearing person

- In bald person, the incision can be placed as far posteriorly as occiput (Fig. 27B).

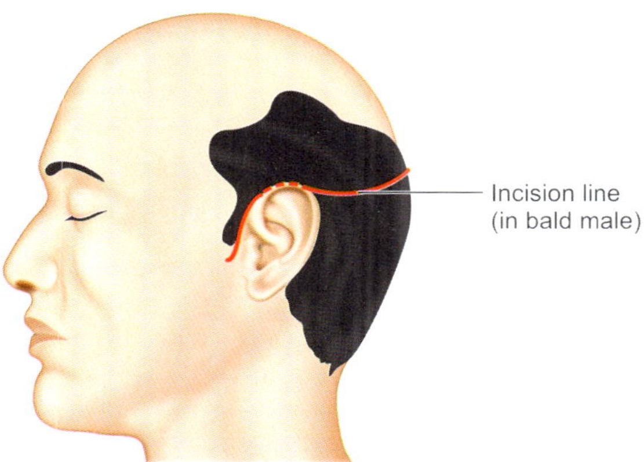

Fig. 27B: Coronal incision in bald person

- Posterior incision does not reduce the access to operative field.

Area to be Accessed

- Depending upon area to be accessed, inferior limit of incision is extended, e.g. if zygomatic arch is to be exposed, a pre- or postauricular extension up to ear lobe is added (Fig. 28).
- If exposure to zygomatic arch and temporomandibular joint is not needed, inferior extent of the incision is not taken and is confined to the helical region.

Design of Incision

There are different alterations in the incisions. These alterations are done to make the scar less noticeable and to achieve accurate reapproximation during closure.

- A simple incision is bow-like incision which is curved in the center.
- Another incision is like a geometric or zigzag pattern (Fig. 29).

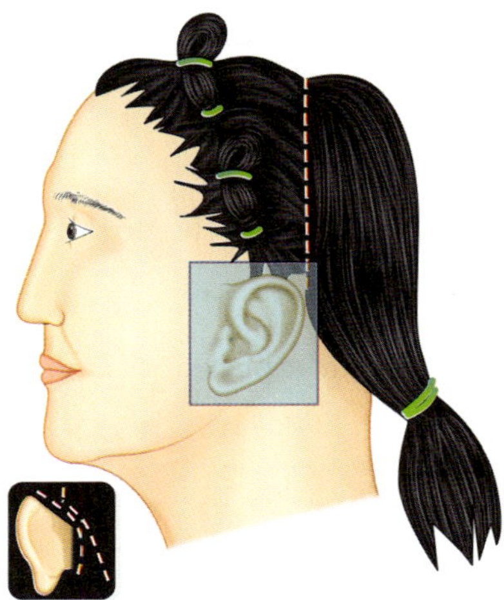

Fig. 28: Postauricular placement of the coronal incision. The incision can be extended into the postauricular sulcus or within the hairline

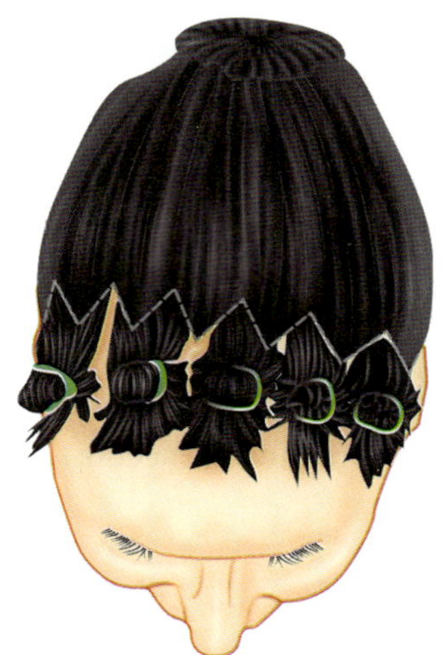

Fig. 29: Geometric or zigzag pattern

Hair Preparation

No preoperative shaving is required. The hairs are parted with comb which helps in positioning the incision. The hairs are treated with chlorhexidine gluconate hand wash, which acts as good hair gel. This allows the hairs to be gathered into clumps, which are secured by elastic bands.

Temporary Tarsorrhaphy

This may be performed with 4-0 monofilament suture with an atraumatic needle. This needle is passed through the gray line of the lids to ensure that some tarsal part is engaged in the sutures so that tearing of eyelid is avoided (Fig. 30).

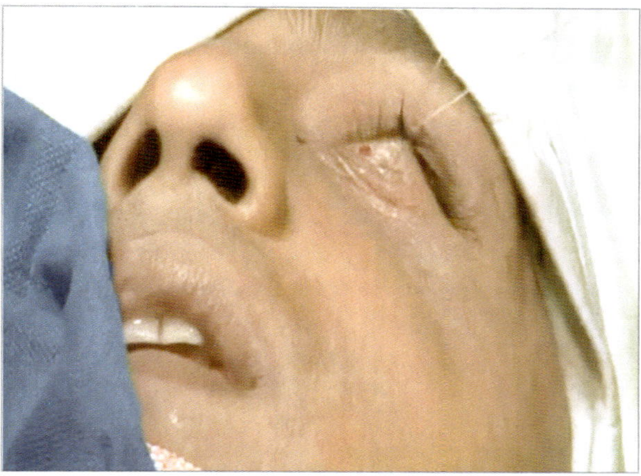

Fig. 30: Temporary tarsorraphy

A small silastic feeding tube is feeded in a suture so that undue pressure is not exerted on delicate skin of eyelid.

Marking of the Incision

- Marking is done with a surgical marker or with methylene blue dye
- Cross hatches are marked properly so that reapproximation is accurate during closure (Fig. 31)

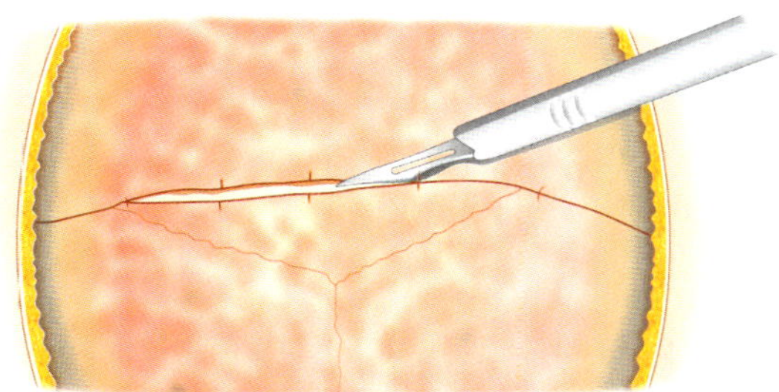

Fig. 31: Well-placed incision line with cross hatches to allow better approximation during closure of the wound

- Some people instead of using cross hatches, uses green needle with ink and it is passed through the scalp ensuring good passage of ink into the tissue
- Initial incision is made from one superior temporal line to other. This is made by a 10 No. blade or bithermic knife.

Hemostasis

There is handsome amount of bleeding during the incision hence several techniques are used to prevent this blood loss (Fig. 32):

- Infiltration with xylocaine 2% with adrenaline (1:200,000) and wait for few minutes
- Use of monopolar or bipolar cautery
- Use of hemostatic clips (Reney's clip) after elevation of wound edge

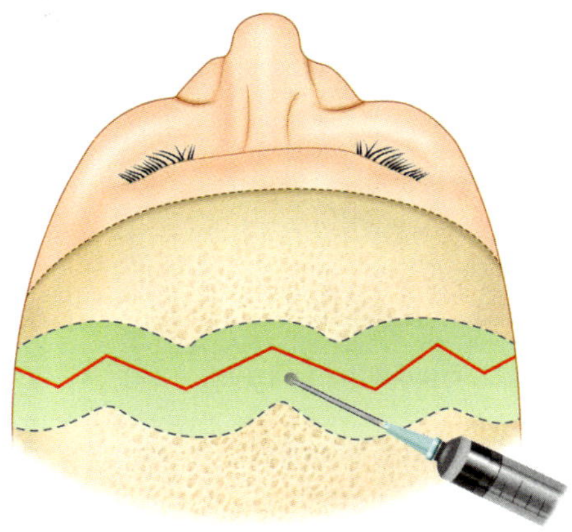

Fig. 32: Hemostatic techniques

- Running mattress sutures are taken along the incision site
- Combination of all these above techniques.

Dissection

- The incision is deepened through the galea to enter the subgaleal space
- The flap is retracted upwards with skin hooks. This gives access to subgaleal layer and helps in further dissection
- The dissection is carried out with diathermy or by scissors according to the surgeon's choice
- As the dissection progress, scalp flap becomes more mobile
- All precautions must be taken so that subperiosteal layer is not damaged.

Lateral Dissection (Temporal Extension of Skin Incision)

The lateral dissection is done with due regards to temporal branch of facial nerve. As the flap is dissected anteroinferiorly, an incision is made in superficial temporalis fascia at an angulation of 45° from base of zygomatic arch to a point, which is at 2.5 cm superior to the lateral orbital margin. This incision is taken with a 15 No. blade. Having made this incision, yellow colored temporal fat pad is seen which separates superficial and deep layers of temporalis fascia. All these exercise is done to prevent injury to temporal branch of facial nerve.

Exposure of Zygoma

- Further dissection is carried inferiorly below the level of superior temporal line keeping close to underlying temporal fascia. This ensures that dissection is beneath the level of temporoparietal fascia, which is a continuation of galea beneath the level of temporal line and It is important as temporal branch of facial nerve runs lateral to the superficial layer of temporalis facia. This dissection is carried out till superior surface of zygomatic arch is reached. Periosteum is sharply incised at the superior aspect of zygomatic arch and then subperiosteal dissection is carried to expose body of zygoma and lateral orbital rim.
- A common complication which can occur is hollowing of temporal fossa area which occurs due to dissection through temporal fat pad. This hollowing can cause significant cosmetic deformity.
- This hollowing is due to fat atrophy, which is caused by devascularization, denervation or displacement of fat pad. In order not to injure this fat pad, dissection should be kept strictly to the lateral surface.

Subperiosteal Exposure of Supraorbital Rim

- Dissection is carried out in subgaleal facial plane up to 3–4 cm superior to supraorbital rim. At around 3 cm above the supraorbital rim, the periosteum is incised from one temporal line to other.
- Further dissection is carried subperiosteally till the supraorbital rim is reached. At this junction, supraorbital neurovascular bundle will be encountered (Fig. 33).
- This simple subperiosteal dissection will allows the bundle to be displaced inferiorly but if there is a true foramen then this bundle needs to be freed by inserting a tip of 5 mm fine osteotome into the foramen and hit inferiorly. This will deliver the inferior border of foramen, freeing the neurovascular bundle. Once the neurovascular bundle is released, a complete subperiosteal resection is done to access orbital roof and medial wall (Fig. 34).

Exposure of Orbital Walls

- Further retraction of the flap inferiorly may be accompalished by subperiostial dissection into the orbit. Dissection of periosteal from

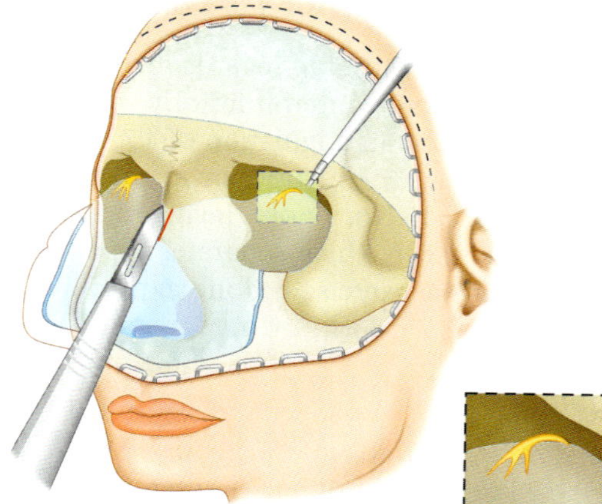

Fig. 33: Relaxing incisions in the sagittal plane through the elevated periosteum over the bridge of the nose are also shown. Use of this technique greatly facilitates dissection more inferiorly along the nasal dorsum

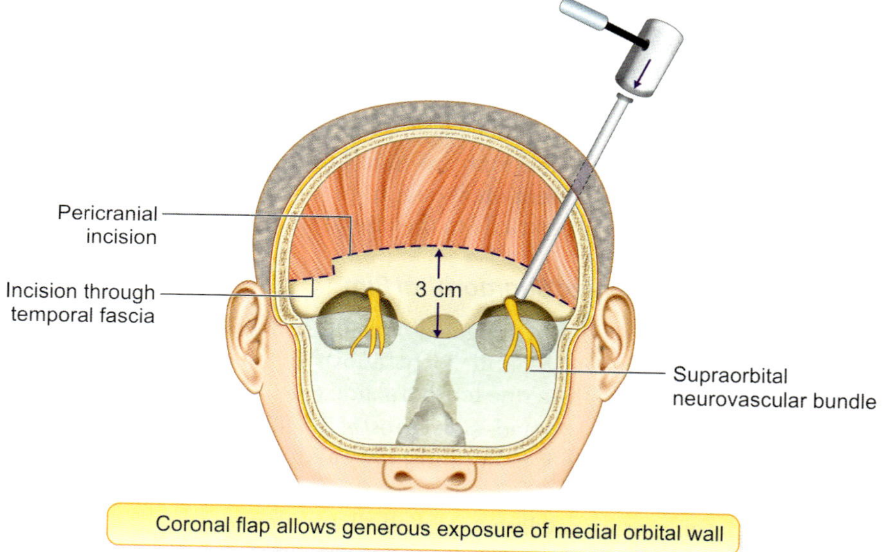

Fig. 34: Technique of removing bone inferior to the supraorbital foramen (when present) so the neurovascular bundle can be released

superior and medial orbital wall releases the flap and allows retraction down to the level of junction of nasal bone and upper lateral cartilage.

- ***Medial orbital wall:*** Subperiosteal dissection is carried in the medial orbital wall. The medial canthal tendon which has two attachments, anterior fibrous and posterior muscular component and is inserted into the anterior and posterior lacrimal crest. The anterior fibrous part of medial canthal tendon is identified and left intact during the course of dissection. This anterior fibrous part is retracted to expose the lacrimal sac. Further dissection is carried out to identify the posterior muscular component of this medial canthal tendon. This tendon is also to be kept intact. Further dissection is carried toward the apex. Following structures will be encounterd during the course of dissection which can be easily remembered by the rule of 24-12-6 which implies the average distance in millimeters from:

- Anterior lacrimal crest to the anterior ethmoidal foramen
- Anterior to posterior ethmoidal foramen
- Posterior ethmoidal foramen to optic canal.

These vessels are cauterized with the help of a bipolar cautery and transaction of vessel may be performed for extended exposure.

- ***Lateral orbital wall:*** The subperiosteal resection is continued over lateral orbital wall. This elevation detaches the lateral canthal tendon which is closely connected over lateral orbital rim and Whitnall tubercle. Dissection deep into the lateral orbital wall exposes the suture line between orbital flank of zygoma and greater wing of sphenoid (spheno- zygomatic suture).
- ***Infraorbital rim and floor of orbit:*** The further subperiosteal dissection is continued medially to expose the infraorbital rim. This dissection is carried till infraorbital foramen and infraorbital nerve. Thus, this approach allows access to lateral part of infraorbital rim and lateral part of floor of orbit.

  To access medial part of orbital floor and rim, one has to take transconjunctival or subciliary incision. This incision is taken prior to coronal incision as there are chances of edema following bicoronal flap elevation.
- ***Exposure of nose:*** Dissection of periostium from medial and superior orbital wall releases the flap and allows retraction down to the level of junction of nasal bone with upper lateral cartilage. The periosteum at the nasofrontal region is carefully incised for further extension. Dissection can be proceeded to expose dorsum and nasal tip (Fig. 35).
- ***Exposure of TM joint and condyle:*** TM joint and ascending ramus of mandible can be exposed with extended coronal incision. This can be done by two maneuvers:

  1. Masseter muscle is cut or released by the help of cautery from its origin along the zygomatic arch and body and then this muscle is stripped from the lateral surface of mandibular ramus to expose ramus, sigmoid notch and coronoid process.
  2. To perform a zygomatic arch osteotomy leaving it pedicled to the masseter muscle. This dissection proceed between bony surface of ramus and underside of muscle.

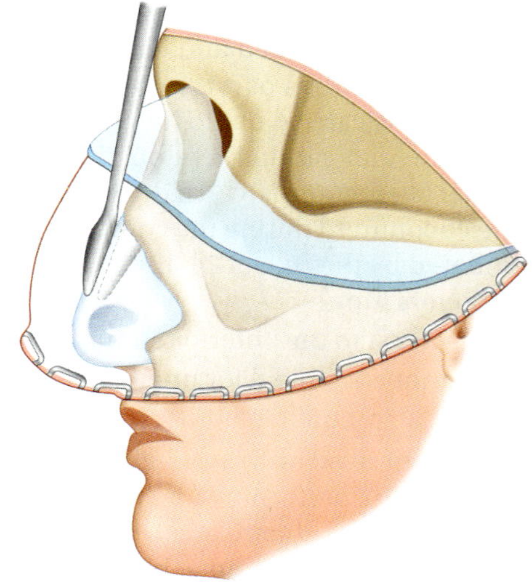

Fig. 35: Dissection inferiorly to the top of the nose with a periosteal elevator

Note: All these exposure hampers, the blood supply and neural supply to the masseter muscle leading to its atrophy. This can cause masseteric dysfunction.

- ***Exposure to temporal fossa:*** This access can be done by stripping the anterior edge of temporalis muscle from temporal surface of zygoma, temporal and frontal bone. The entire temporalis muscle can be stripped subperiostealy from temporal fossa, if necessary. Utmost care should be taken to preserve vascular supply of temporalis muscle.

Pericranial Flap

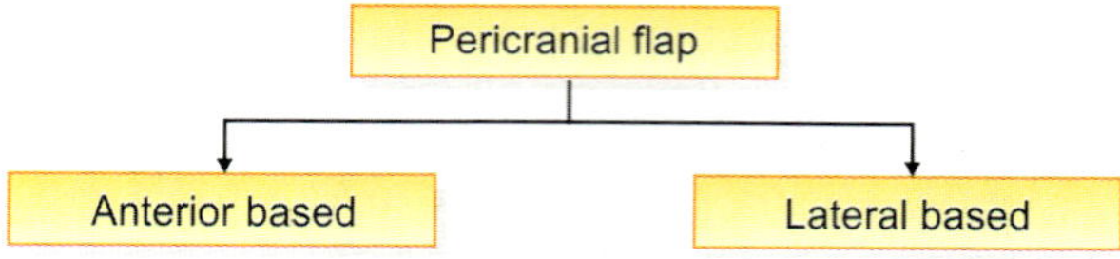

Indications

- In cases of frontal sinus repair
- In cases of anterior skull base repair
- Sealing of nasal cavity.

This pericranial flap take its supply from deep branch of superior orbital and supratrochlear artery. These vessels lies between galea and pericranium so to prevent devascularization of the flap, dissection is carried subperiostially. If subgaleal dissection is carried, this should not be continued inferiorly toward supraorbital rim.

Anteriorly-based Pericranial Flaps

- Anteriorly-based pericranial flaps are most commonly taken. To develop a large rectangular flap, incision through the pericranium are made bilaterally along the superior temporal line. Pericranium is loosely adherent to the bone, so it can be easily raised with the help of periosteal elevator. After dissection of forehead and supraorbital region, the area of flap increases (Fig. 36).

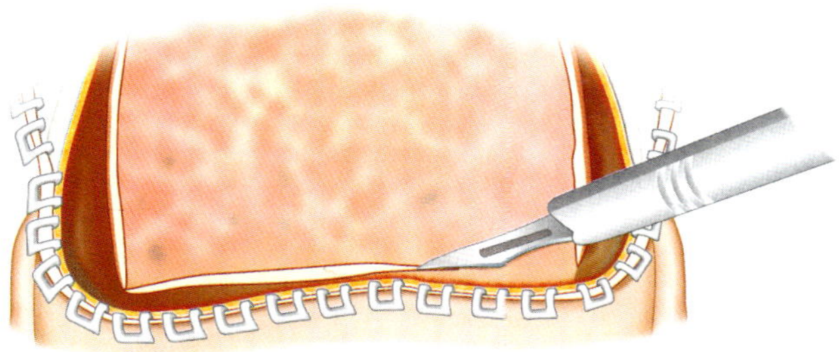

Fig. 36: Pericranial incision

Laterally-based Pericranial Flaps

- Laterally-based flaps are taken in cases of trauma where viability of anterior-based flap is in question. Too laterally-based flap may be raised with blood supply coming from the lateral aspect. The subperiosteal resection allows reflection of flap inferior to superior and lateral orbital margin.

HARVESTING CRANIAL BONE GRAFT (FIG. 37)

The advantage of this cranial flap is a large stock of cranial bone graft can be harvested. Incision through the periosteum exposes this bone. Normally, the graft is harvested from the parietal bone area. The graft should be taken from the skull over nondominant hemisphere. The harvesting area should be 1.5 cm away from the suture line to prevent injury to the sagittal sinus. This bone has three tables:

1. Outer table
2. Inner table
3. Middle table (diploic layer).

Even harvesting the outer table can be associated with potential intracranial morbidities. With the help of burrs and flexible osteotomes, the require area of bone is harvested. Either outer cortex is taken after splitting through the diploic layer from the inner table or full thickness bone graft can be taken. In that case, the inner table is used as harvested bone and the outer table is replaced back on the skull.

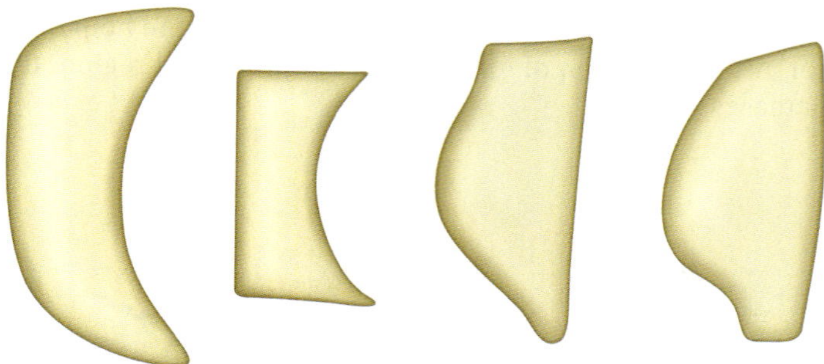

Fig. 37: Various shape of cranial bone graft harvested

In cases of defect, it can be filled with bone graft or titanium mesh. A low profile plates or screw are used to replace the outer table or to secure the titanium mesh.

Bone dust and bone patties can be harvested in copious amount by running a drill in a very low speed over this bone.

CLOSURE

- Closure should be done in following sequence:
- Bone graft
- Pericranium
- Lateral canthal ligament
- Temporalis muscle
- Superficial temporal fascia
- Skin.

Lateral Canthopexy

If lateral canthus attachment is detached, it needs to be reanchored. A suture is passed through the lateral canthal tendon and then passed through the hole of lateral orbital wall and then again passed through the temporalis fascia and then secured.

Refixation of Temporalis Muscle

If temporalis muscle is elevated from temporal surface of the orbit, it should be resutured to the soft tissue cuff left along the superior temporal line.

Suturing of Temporalis Fascia

The incised temporalis fascia is resutured by slow absorbing sutures (Fig. 38).

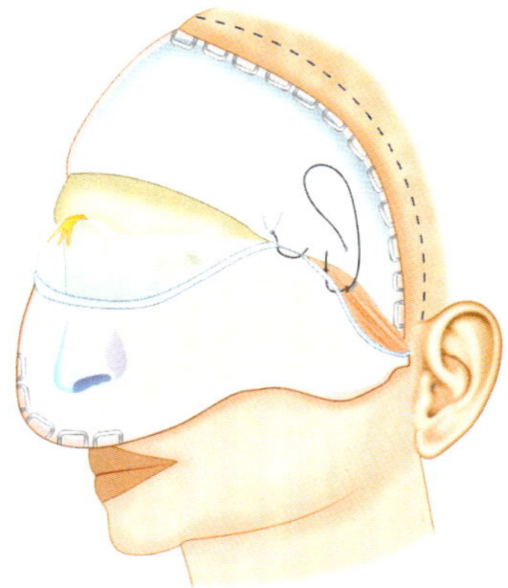

Fig. 38: Suturing the superficial layer of the temporalis fascia. Note that the inferior edge of fascia is sutured to more superior location that the cut superior edge

Drain Placement

Drain is placed and brought out from the scalp, posterior to the incision.

Skin Closure

Skin is closed in three layers:

1. For galea, 2-0 vicryl is used
2. Skin is sutured with non-absorbable sutures or stapled.
3. Preauricular extension, if taken needs to closed in layers.

Dressing

Head dressing is given to prevent hematoma formation. Care must be taken that this dressing should not be too tight as this can increase the periorbital edema.

ZYGOMATICOFRONTAL SUTURE

Brow Incision

This is the most commonly used technique.

Advantages

- Extremely low complication rate
- No special expertise required.

Disadvantages

- Scar with fair aesthetic results
- Localized hair loss can occur.

Steps

1. *Incision*: Incision is taken with 15 number blade through the skin at the superior border of lateral brow over the zygomaticofrontal suture line (Figs 39 and 40).

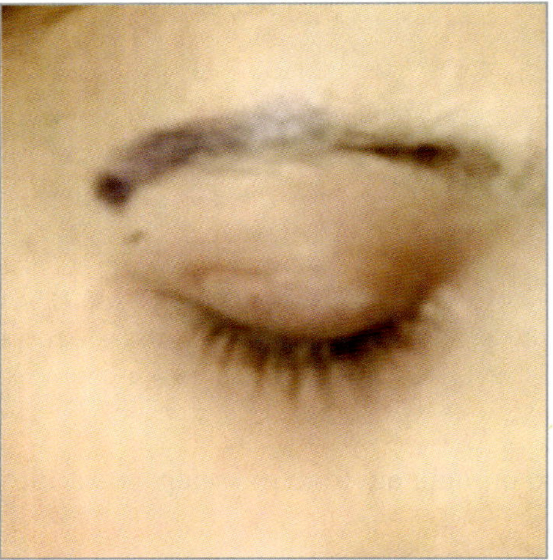

Fig. 39: Marking of brow incision

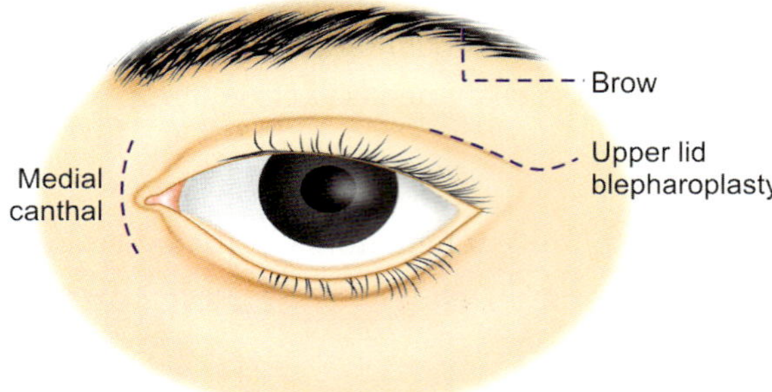

Fig. 40: Schematic marking for various incisions used to expose ZF suture

   - This incision is parallel to hair shaft.
2. *Dissection*: Blunt dissection is carried out through muscle fibers till periosteum is rached—periosteum is sharply cut.

- Fracture is reduced and fixed
- After reduction and fixation of fracture, periosteum is reapproximated
- Wound is closed in layers.

UPPER LID BLEPHAROPLASTY APPROACH (FIG. 41)

Advantages

- Gives excellent access to frontozygomatic suture
- Good aesthetic results.

Steps

1. *Incision:* Incision is placed at upper lid skin crease from midpupil to lateral orbital rim.

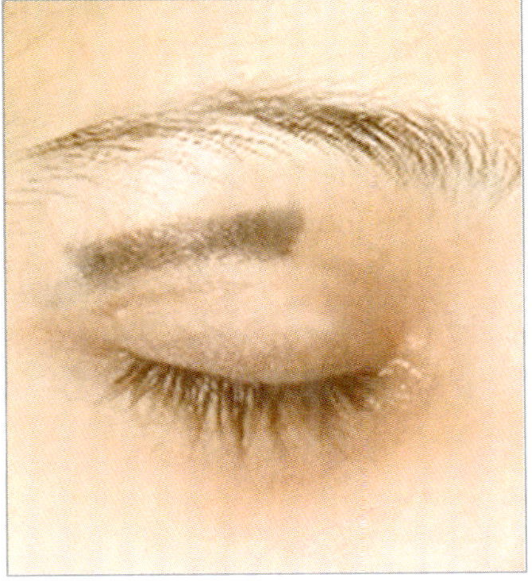

Fig. 41: Marking for upper lid blepharoplasty incision

   - There are chances of bleeding. Hemostasis is achieved with bipolar cautery. Avoid use of monopolar cautery as this can damage the underlying sclera because of thermal conduction.
2. *Dissection*: The dissection is carried out above orbital septa towards zygomaticofrontal suture:
   - The periosteum is incised and fracture is exposed (Fig. 42)

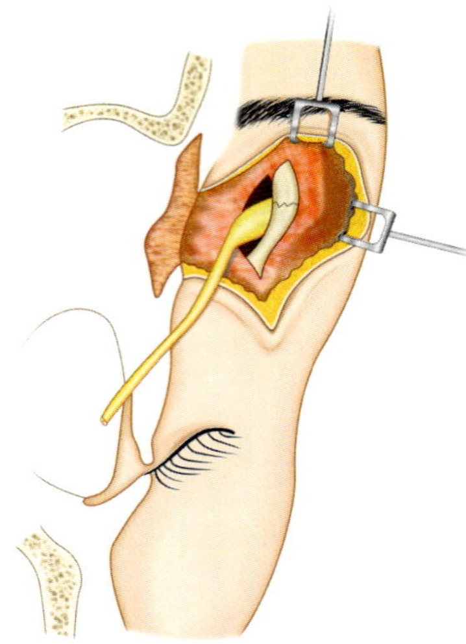

Fig. 42: Schematic picture showing upper lid blepharoplasty approach to expose the ZF suture line

- Fracture is reduced and fixed
- After reduction and fixation of fracture the periosteum is reapproximated
- Skin is closed by running intracutaneous or mattress sutures without subcutaneous sutures.

CHAPTER

Approaches to Maxilla Fracture

Maxilla is 2nd largest bone of the face. Each maxillary bone contributes in the formation of (Fig. 1):

1. Nose
2. Orbit
3. Alveolus
4. Palate
5. Infratemporal and pterygopalatine fossa

   Each maxillary bone have (Fig. 2):

   a. A body
   b. Four processes
      1. Frontal
      2. Zygomatic
      3. Alveolar
      4. Palatine

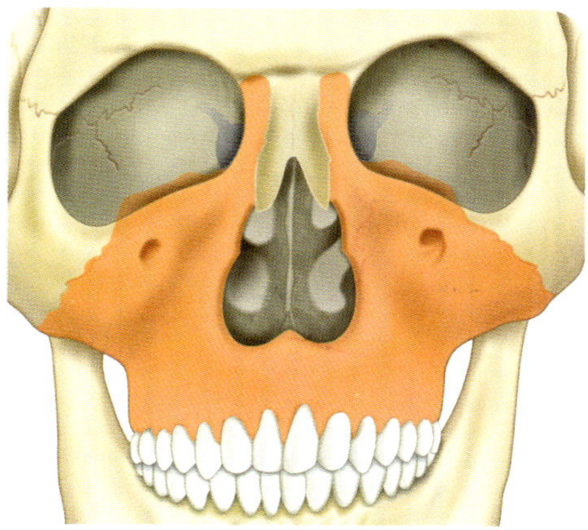

Fig. 1: Contribution of maxillary bone to facial skeleton

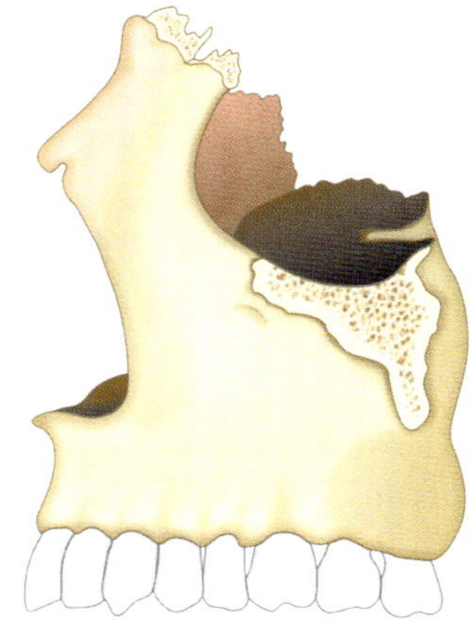

Fig. 2: Body and various processes of maxilla

MAXILLA FRACTURE

To deal with different levels of Le Fort fractures, following approaches are used, individually or in combination. The approaches are:

Intraoral Approach (Maxillary Vestibular Approach)

It can be approached by:

1. Gingivobuccal sulcus incision (sublabial incisional) (Fig. 3).
2. Marginal gingival incision (sulcular incision) (Fig. 3).

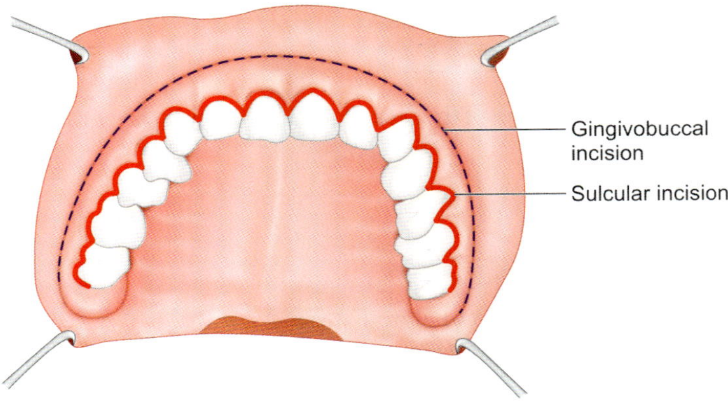

Fig. 3: Dotted line shows gingivobuccal sulcus incision while dark continuous incision mark shows sulcular incision

Gingivobuccal Sulcus Incision (Sublabial Incision)

This is a typical incision which we use for Caldwell Luc procedures. It can be done under local anesthesia.

Areas exposed with this incision are:

- Infraorbital rim area
- Lateral buttress of maxilla
- Maxillary zygomatic buttress.

Advantages

- No external scar is seen
- It is an intraoral approach.

Disadvantages

- Chances of wound dehiscence
- Chances of wound infection and increased chances of scar formation.

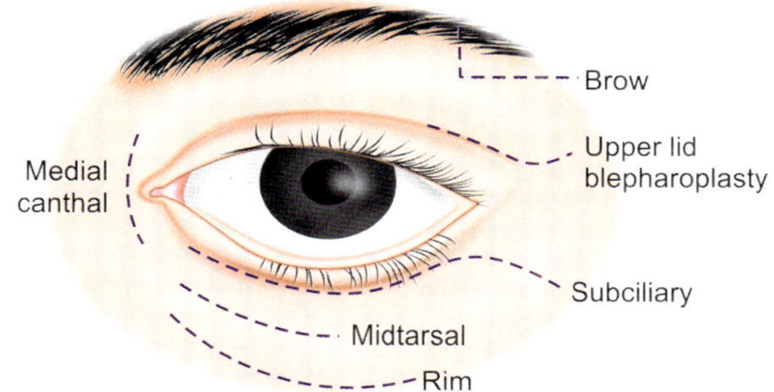

Fig. 4: Incisions used for approaching various processes of maxilla

Steps

- Incision is taken over mucosa 4 to 5 mm beyond the level of attached gingiva
- Infiltration is done at the incision site
- Dissection is carried out till the periosteum of maxilla is seen
- Fracture site is exposed, reduced and fixed
- Wound is closed in layers.

Marginal Gingival Incision (Sulcular Incision)

Advantages

- Minimal scar formation
- Less chances of infection
- Wound dehiscence is never seen with this approach.

Steps

- Incision is taken along the attached gingival margin
- Dissection is similar as before
- Wound is closed in layers. Suture is passed through teeth as intermaxillary fixation.

Lower Eyelid Approach (Fig. 4)

Areas exposed with this approach are:
- Infraorbital rim
- Orbital floor
- Upper part of maxillary buttress.

A detail of this approach is mentioned in approaches to orbit.

Upper Lid Blepharoplasty Approach

This approach gives excellent access to frontozygomatic suture.

Advantages

- Good esthetic results
- Excellent exposure for manipulation.

Steps

- It is done under general anesthesia
- After tarsorrhaphy has been done, an incision is placed in upper lid skin crease from midpupil to lateral orbital rim. Hemostasis is achieved with cauterization
- Skin muscle flap is elevated above the septum. This dissection is carried toward frontozygomatic suture
- Periosteum is incised with the help of 15 number blade. Fracture area is exposed
- After reduction of fracture, wound is closed in layers.

BROW INCISION

This is the most commonly used technique.

Advantages

- Extremely low complication rate
- No expertise required.

Disadvantages

- Scar with fair esthetic results
- Localized hair loss can occur.

Steps

Incision

Incision is taken with 15 number blade through the skin at the superior border of lateral brow over the zygomaticofrontal suture line.

This incision is parallel to hair shaft.

Dissection

- Blunt dissection is carried out through muscle fibers till periosteum is reached
- Periosteum is sharply cut
- Fracture is reduced and fixed
- After reduction and fixation of fracture the periosteum is reapproximated
- Wound is closed in layers.

Coronal Approach (Fig. 5)

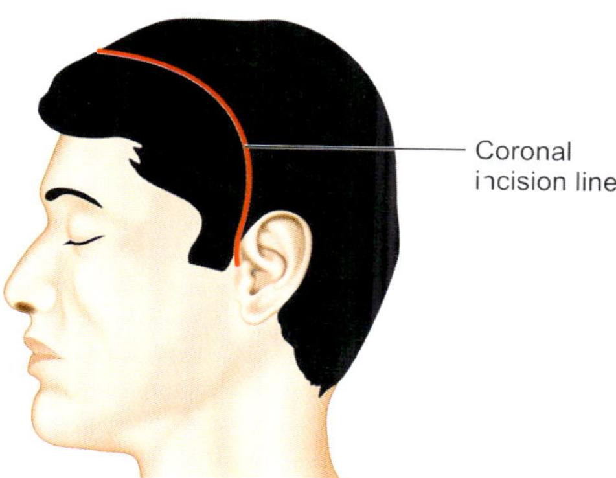

Fig. 5: Coronal incision used to deal panfacial fractures

- This approach requires extensive dissection
- It is commonly used in cases of multiple facial fractures
  - The principle and steps have been described in Chapter 7, "Approaches to Zygomatic Fracture".

CHAPTER

Approaches to Orbital Fracture

SURGICAL APPROACHES TO ORBITAL FRACTURES

Orbital trauma is divided into:

1. Isolated orbital wall fracture.
2. Orbital wall fracture associated with globe injuries.

Any patient of orbital trauma should first go through an ophthalmic checkup which needs to be done by an ophthalmologist.

Orbital wall fracture is broadly divided into four types:

a. Inferior wall fracture
    i. Inferior orbital rim fractures
    ii. Orbital floor fractures.
b. Superior wall fracture—it separates orbit from brain and is rare in nature.
c. Lateral wall fracture—it is formed by the zygoma bone.
d. Medial wall fracture—consists of thin lamina papyracea which separates nose from orbit.

ORBITAL FLOOR FRACTURE

Options Available for Treatment of Orbital Floor Fracture

1. Conservative approach.
2. Surgical approach
    a. Open approach
    b. Endoscopic approach.

Indications for Surgery

- Persistent diplopia after 10–14 days of trauma with a positive force duction test

- Radiological confirmation of an orbital floor fracture with entrapment of the inferior rectus or perimuscular tissues surrounding the inferior rectus.

KEY POINTS

- Diplopia may be present initially after trauma but may resolve as the neuropraxia and/or orbital edema subside
- A subclass of orbital fracture with entrapment is called *white-eye fracture* in children. These patients need to be treated early
- Enophthalmos of greater than 2 mm persisting for 10–14 days after trauma is cosmetically significant and therefore an indication for surgery. Orbital edema that is present initially may mask the exact severity of enophthalmos. Therefore, measurements must be rechecked once the orbital edema has subsided
- Fractures involving one-third or more of the orbit need to be repaired. If left unattended, these fractures tend to result in significant enophthalmos. When surgery is indicated, it is usually best performed as close to 2 weeks from the date of trauma. This allows the swelling to subside and a more accurate examination of the orbit can be performed

Indications for Endoscopic Repair of Orbital Floor Fracture

- Patient with trap door fracture and medial blowout fracture are excellent candidates for endoscopic repair (Figs 1A and B).

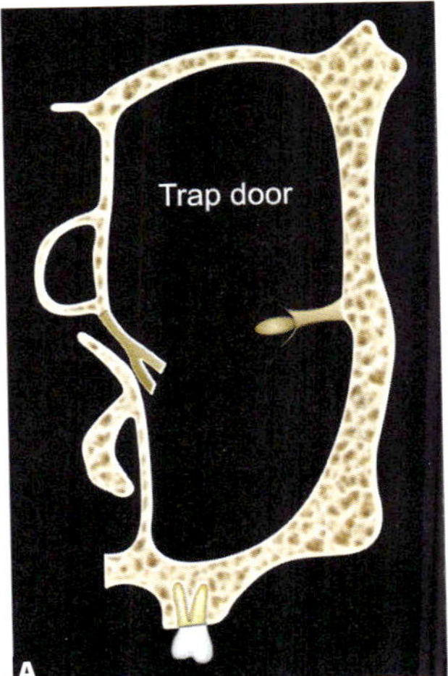

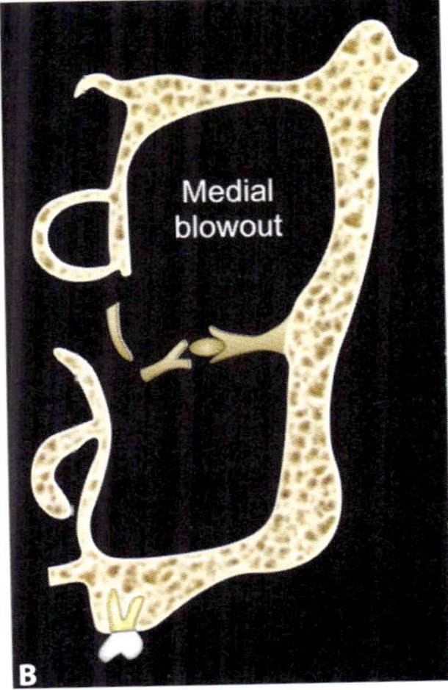

Figs 1A and B: (A) Trap door fracture where fracture segment is hinged at one end; (B) Medial blowout fracture where fracture is extending to medial wall but not extending beyond inferior orbital nerve

Preoperative Evaluation

- Short history of mode of injury should be taken
- Ophthalmic evaluation should be undertaken to avoid any visual loss from optic neuropathy, retinal detachment or hyphema
- Computed tomography (CT) scan of orbit needs to be done to see the extent of floor injury and accompanying injuries. A cut of minimum 1 mm is required (Prolapsed fat and entrapment of muscle should be seen)
- Head injury and spine injury should be ruled out. Patient needs to be hemodynamically stable prior to surgery.

Surgical Steps

- Repair is normally done in general anesthesia. Patient is placed in supine position (head high position of around 30°)
- The forced duction test should be performed to determine ocular motility immediately after general anesthesia is induced
- Two percent lignocaine with adrenaline is infiltrated sublabially
- A 4 cm incision is made in gingivobuccal sulcus (Fig. 2), ensuring adequate mucosal stump at the alveolar end, so that suturing is convenient.
- Incision is deepened through the periosteum to reach the anterior wall of maxilla. The periosteum is elevated exposing the anterior wall of maxilla up to the level of infraorbital nerve (Fig. 3)

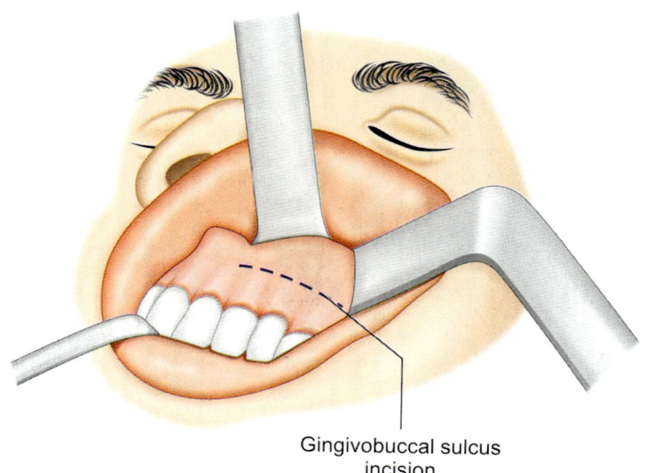

Fig. 2: Adequate length (4–5 cm) of incision is made few mm away from attached gingival margin

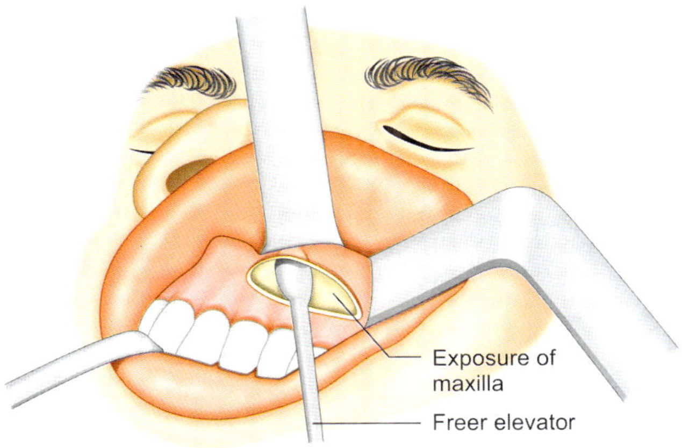

Fig. 3: Dissection carried out in subperiosteal plane to expose the maxillary bone

- Care is taken to avoid excessive traction or trauma to nerve. With the help of an osteotome and Kerrison punch, appropriate sized window is created in thin wall of maxilla (Fig. 4).

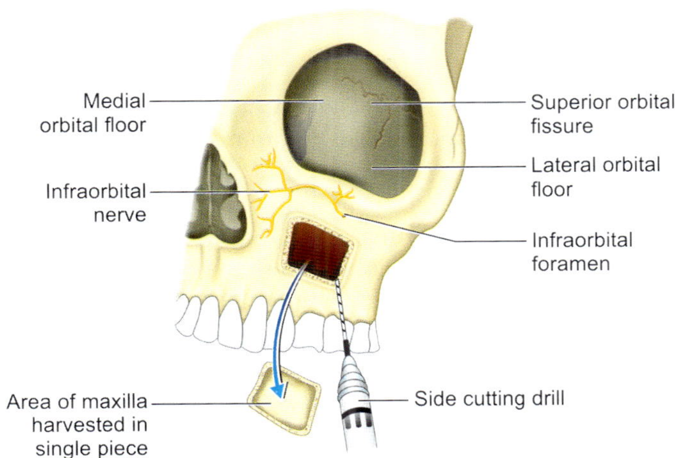

Fig. 4: Appropriate sized bony window is made over anterior face of maxilla to access floor of the orbit

- Lip is retracted and a cottonoid/patty soaked in 4% lignocaine and adrenaline is placed in maxillary sinus for decongestion of mucosa
- Then the endoscope is introduced to inspect the orbital floor. Any defect in orbital floor is analyzed for size, location, soft tissue prolapse and entrapment

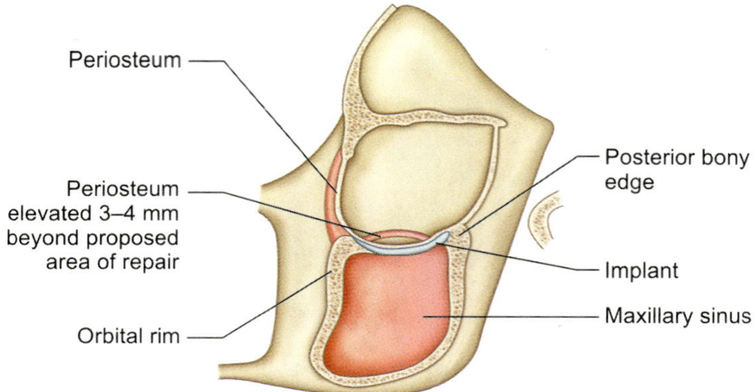

Fig. 5: Prolapsed tissue is reduced back to the orbit and a titanium mesh/implant is placed to repair the floor

- Any entrapped tissue is made free and is reduced back to orbit with the help of freer's elevator (Fig. 5).

Hinge Fracture (Fig. 1A)

- Any hinge fracture after replacement of soft tissues to orbit is then allowed to snap back into place maintaining the reduction
- Excessive medial dissection is avoided as this may destabilize the hinge and may require placement of implant.

Medial Blowout Fracture (Fig. 1B)

- Elevate the mucosa around defect and expose the edge
- Orbital content is reduced and all comminuted fragments of bone are removed
- Size of defect is assessed and suitable implant is trimmed to size, which is 1 mm bigger than size of defect
- Implant is inserted over the stable posterior edge and is directed toward anterior edge with the help of freer elevator and suction
- During the manipulation, constant check needs to be kept that implant at posterior end is not shifted and remains at the same position
- Anterior edge and the posterior edge form the primary area of support
- Pulse test (gentle external pressure is applied at globe and the pulsations are observed through the endoscope) is performed to see whether implant is stable. Forced duction test is performed again to check any restriction of movement.

Precautions

- Injuries to maxillary mucosa should be avoided
- Injuries to infraorbital nerve should be avoided
- No bony fragment is pushed into orbital cavity

- Any bone fragment or mucosa overhanging at area of maxillary ostium should be removed to prevent infection
- Bone chip of anterior wall can be fixed again or kept open
- Wound is closed in layers by 3.0 vicryl suture
- Failure to repair the fracture endoscopically will necessitate an alternative approach—subciliary and transconjunctival approach.

OPEN METHODS

A. Skin Incision

1. Subciliary incision (standard and converse incision).
2. Midtarsal incision.
3. Infraorbital rim incision.

Anatomic Considerations

The different layers of lower eyelid are:
- Skin
- Subcutaneous tissue
- Orbicularis oculi muscle
- Orbital septum
- Orbital fat
- Inferior tarsal muscle
  - Isolated skin flap should not be used as it is a random flap. Elevation of this skin flap can lead to infarction of skin and there are increased chances of vertical lid shortening leading to scleral show and ectropion
  - Always skin muscle flap has to be used as there are fewer chances of vertical lid shortening and scleral show
  - The orbital septa of lower eyelid is a continuation of mucoperiosteum layer of maxilla which lies in between orbicularis muscle and orbital fat. Its lower ends are attached few mm below orbital rim
  - All precautions have to be taken to prevent breach in orbital septum to prevent prolapse of orbital fat
  - Incision in infraorbital rim periosteum is taken few mm below the rim to prevent injury to orbital septa.

Subciliary Incision

Standard Subciliary Incision (Figs 6A to D)

Steps

- Incision is taken 2 to 3 mm below the eyelashes and extended only 8 to 10 mm lateral to lateral canthus

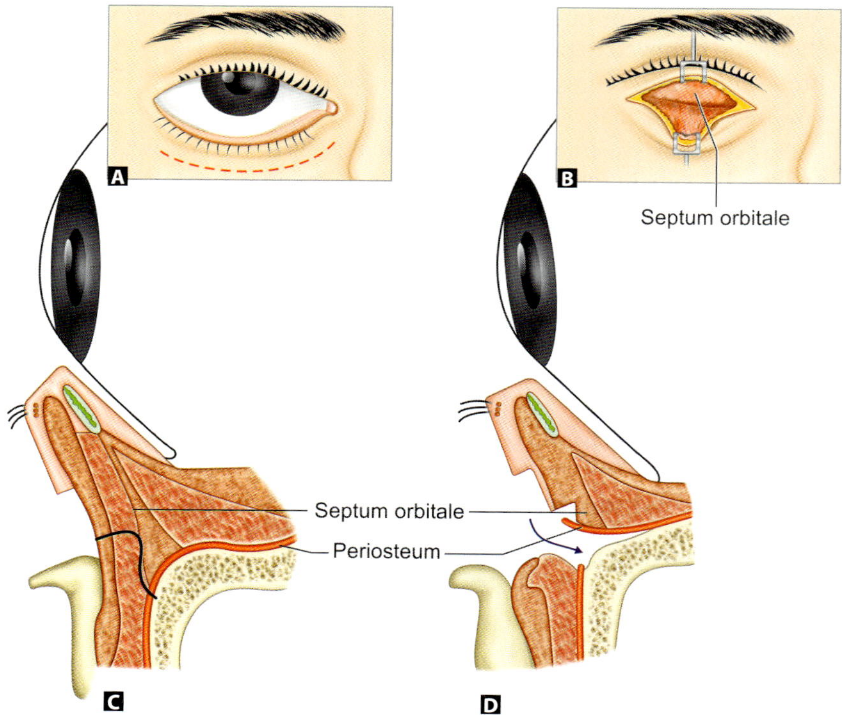

Figs 6A to D: Subciliary incision: (A) marking of incision few mm below the eyelashes; (B) Elevation of the myocutaneous flap; (C) Incision over the periosteum below the attachment of orbital septum; (D) Exposure of the orbital rim

- Avoid extension of this incision into cheek as this leads to noticeable scar
- Skin muscle flap is elevated till the infraorbital rim is reached
- Utmost care is taken to prevent injury to orbital septa
- At infraorbital rim, periosteum is incised few mm below the infraorbital rim to prevent injury to orbital septa
- This periosteum is elevated along with rim and continued over floor of orbit
- Orbital contents are retracted with special retractor to expose orbital floor area (Contents of orbit are reduced and a mesh is placed)
- The periosteal edge of the incision can be marked with fine silk suture and cut short on each side to identify the edge of closure.

Disadvantages

- Highest incidence of lid retraction
- Increased chances of scleral show
- Increased chances of ectropion.

Converse Subciliary Incision (Fig. 7)

Steps

- The incision is taken 2 to 3 mm below the eyelashes
- Only skin flap is elevated for few mm thus resecting superficial to tarsal orbicularis muscle and preventing injury to the same
- Below the tarsal plate incision is taken over the orbicularis muscle thus raising the skin muscle flap till infraorbital rim
- This incision prevents injury to orbicularis oculi part of tarsal plate thus reducing chances of ectropion and lid retraction
- At infraorbital rim the periosteum is incised few mm below the infraorbital rim to prevent injury to orbital septa. This periosteum is elevated along with rim and continued over floor of orbit

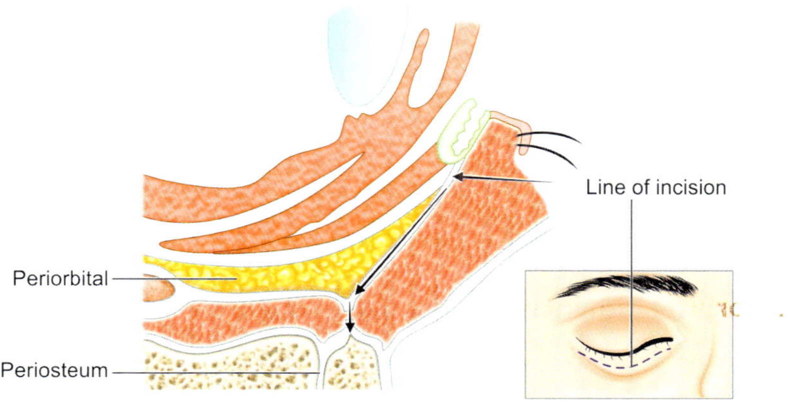

Fig. 7: Showing converse subciliary incision wherein skin flap is elevated for few mm and then skin muscle flap is elevated

- Orbital content is retracted with special retractor to expose orbital floor area. Content of orbit is reduced and a mesh is placed
- The periosteal edge of the incision can be marked with fine silk suture and cut short on each side to identify the edge of closure.

Midtarsal Incision (Fig. 8)

- Incision is taken at the lower eyelid crease (1 mm below the midtarsal crease in the lid)
- Skin muscle flap is elevated
- Rest of the dissection is similar to subciliary approach.

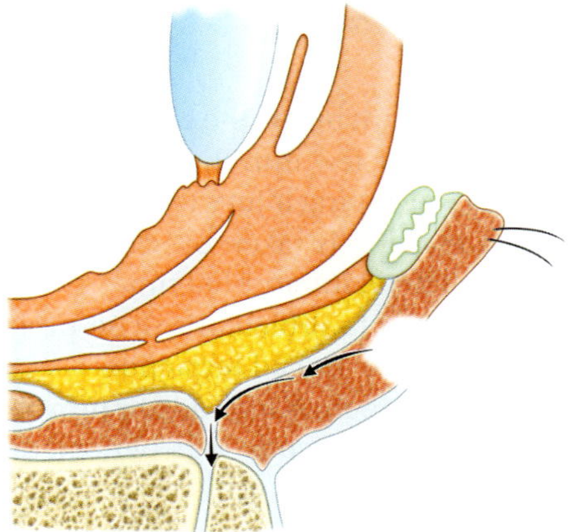

Fig. 8: Midtarsal incision

Advantages

This incision does not denervate the pretarsal orbicularis occuli muscle leading to less chance of ectropion and scleral show.

Disadvantages

Scar is more visible than subciliary incision.

Infraorbital Rim Incision (Fig. 9)

- Incision is taken directly on infraorbital rim.

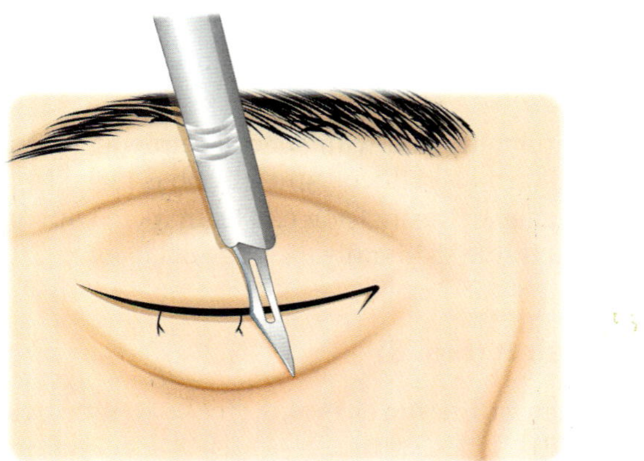

Fig. 9: Showing infraorbital rim incision

Disadvantages

This incision gives very bad scar.

B. Conjunctival Incision (Fig. 10)

Also called as inferior fornix incision.

Advantages

- No scar is seen leading to best cosmetic result
- Lower incidence of ectropion
- Less changes of lid shortening
- Healing is faster
- Rapid procedure as no skin and muscle dissection is required.

Disadvantages

- Restricted access
- Limited extension due to presence of lacrimal sac system
- Greater degree of operative dexterity is required, if complications have to be avoided.

Two Types of Conjunctival Approaches

1. Preseptal
2. Retroseptal
   - Retroseptal approach is more direct and easier to perform than preseptum approach
   - These approaches are named according to dissection performed in relation to septa

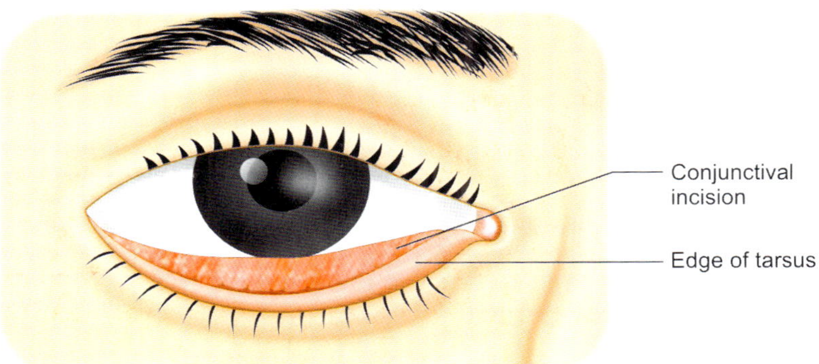

Fig. 10: Conjunctival inc sion

- Retroseptal approach has chances of encountering periorbital fat which hardly cause any ill effect.

Conjunctival approach can be extended laterally by doing lateral canthotomy and inferior cantholysis if need of surgery demand for sake of exposure.

Incision

Once the lower lid is everted, note the position of the lower tarsal plate through the conjunctiva.

Blunt-tipped pointed scissors are used to dissect through the small incision over the conjunctiva inferiorly toward the infraorbital rim.

The traction sutures are used to evert the lower eyelid during the dissection.

Dissection

Spread the scissors to clear a pocket just posterior to the orbital septum, ending posterior to the orbital rim. Scissors are used to incise the conjunctiva and lower lid retractors midway between the inferior margin of the tarsal plate and the inferior conjunctival fornix thus flap is created till inferior orbital rim (Fig. 11).

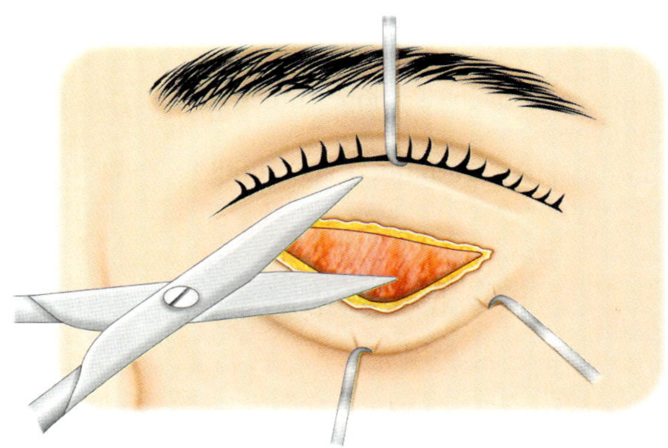

Fig. 11: Flap created just posterior to orbital septum

Incision on Inferior Orbital Periosteum

Incision is taken few mm below the inferior orbital rim. Periosteum is elevated and dissection of periosteum is continued along the floor of orbit. Incised edge of periosteum is tied with ligature, so that it can be identified easily during closure. A broad malleable retractor should be placed as soon as feasible to protect the orbit and to confine any herniating periorbital fat and expose floor area.

Closure

Periosteal sutures are not absolutely necessary, but if exposure permits, they can be placed. The conjunctiva is closed with a running 6-0 chromic gut suture. The ends of the suture may be buried.

No attempt is made to re-approximate the lower lid retractors because they are intimately in contact with the conjunctiva and will be adequately repositioned with closure of that layer.

A 4-0 silk or other long lasting suture is used to reattach the lateral portion of the inferior tarsal plate to the superior portion of the canthal tendon and surrounding tissues. It is important that this suture be securely placed in the appropriate location or the lateral canthal area will never appear normal. When the inferior limb of the canthal tendon is severed during the approach, only a minute amount of canthal tendon remains attached to the lower tarsus. Therefore, the canthopexy suture can be placed through the lateral border of the tarsus if the tendon attached is insufficient to hold a suture. It is easier to pass the suture through the lateral border of the lower tarsus and/or cut portion of the lateral canthal tendon if the skin is dissected slightly from them.

This is very easily performed by taking a number 15 scalpel and incising between the tarsus and the skin.

A cleavage plane exists in this location, and the tissue readily separates. The tarsus is grasped with forceps and a suture is passed through either the cut tendon or the lateral border of the tarsus in such a fashion that a firm bit of tissue is engaged. Once a good bite of lower tarsus has been taken with the suture, the suture needle should be placed through the superior limb of the lateral canthal tendon.

The bulk of the lateral canthal tendon attaches to the orbital tubercle, 3 to 4 mm *posterior* to the orbital margin. Following canthotomy, the superior limb of the canthal tendon is still attached to the orbital tubercle. It is important to place the suture as deep behind the orbital rim as possible to adapt the lower eyelid to the globe. If the suture is not properly placed, the eyelid will not contact the globe laterally, giving an unnatural appearance. Therefore, the suture needle should pass very far posteriorly and superiorly to ensure that it grasps the superior limb of the tendon. An effective method to pass this suture is to identify the superior limb of the canthal tendon first with small, toothed forceps placed into the incision. The forceps are passed along the medial side of the lateral orbital rim for a few mm until the dense fibers of the superior limb are located. While the tendon is held, the suture needle is passed through the tendon. The surgeon should pull on the two ends of the suture to enclosure that the suture is firmly attached to ligamentous tissue. The suture is then tied, with the lower lid drawn into position. Finally, subcutaneous sutures and 6-0 skin suture are placed along the horizontal lateral canthotomy.

Approaches to Medial Wall of the Orbit

Medial wall fractures are less common than blowout fractures. These fractures are underappreciated in their incidence and importance. Because of this under appreciation, incidences of delayed enophthalmos are reported frequently.

1. External
2. Endoscopic.

External

a. Subciliary incision
b. Conjunctival
c. Direct medial canthal approach
d. Medial brow incision
e. Upper eyelid crease incision
f. Coronal incision.

Endoscopic

a. Transcaruncular approach
b. Intranasal or endonasal approach.

Indications of Medial Wall Fracture Repair

Minimal displacement of medial wall fracture with no signs of herniation of orbital content and minimal enophthalmos are treated conservatively.

Surgical intervention is required if there is:

- Persistent symptomatic diplopia
- Positive force duction test with clear evidence of medial rectus muscle entrapment on CT scan
- Large defect of more than 50% of medial wall likely to cause secondary enophthalmos
- Early enophthalmos of more than 2 mm
- Pain during horizontal eye movement.

External approaches like subciliary and conjunctival incisions give more exposure to the orbital floor area and additionally some part of anterior and inferior part of medial orbital wall. Details of these approaches have already been described in the management of floor fracture.

Direct Medial Canthal Approach

Advantages

Used to access medial and inferomedial aspect of orbit.

Disadvantages

- Obvious external scar
- Chances of web formation
- Risk of telecanthus due to detachment of medial canthal tendon.

Medial Brow Approach

Disadvantages

- Limited access to anterior and superior aspect of medial orbital wall
- There may be a failure in attempt to free intact medial rectus muscle from posterior medial wall fracture because of its close proximity to orbital nerve.

Lid Crease Incision

Advantages

Cosmetically good but limitations are same as medial brow incision.

Coronal Approach

Again this approach is indicated in cases of medial orbital wall fracture with fracture of adjacent structures like nasoethmoid, zygoma and frontal bone.

Disadvantages

- External scar
- Alopecia
- Injury to branches of 7th nerve
- Extensive surgical resection
- Loss hospital stay.

ENDOSCOPIC APPROACHES

Transcaruncular

- Surgery is performed under GA
- Infiltration is done with xylocaine 2% + adrenaline (1:200,000) into medial conjunctiva using a fine needle

- Two parallel traction sutures are placed in medial conjunctiva posterior to caruncle with 4-0 silk
- These tractional sutures facilitate in incision placement
- A corneal sheath is used to protect the cornea from damage from surgical instruments
- A slight curvilinear incision around 1 cm is taken between 2 sutures.

Resection

- With the help of a blunt scissor, further dissection is carried out toward the medial orbital wall immediately posterior to the lacrimal sac
- Blunt dissection is then carried out to incise the periorbita just behind the posterior lacrimal crest and medial orbital wall is exposed
- The periorbita is further elevated superiorly, inferiorly and posteriorly by freer's elevator thereby creating a periosteal opening which is wider than the conjunctival incision
- An *optical cavity* is created and maintained with the help of retractors. Baby retractors are inserted medially and narrow malleable retractors are put laterally to pull the orbital content laterally.

Surgical Anatomy

Anterior ethmoidal artery lies 24 mm away from anterior lacrimal crest and posterior ethmoidal vessel lies 36 mm away from anterior lacrimal crest and optic nerve lies 7 mm behind the posterior ethmoidal artery.

Use of Endoscope

- A 2.5 mm endoscope is introduced through the optical cavity which is retracted with the help of retractors and further dissection is carried out
- Utmost care is taken in the area of anterior ethmoidal artery. This anterior ethmoidal artery can be cauterized, if required with the help of bipolar cautery
- Then further dissection is carried posteriorly up to posterior ethmoidal vessels which indicates limit of safe dissection on medial wall
- A horizontal line connecting anterior to posterior ethmoidal vessels indicates superior limit of ethmoid sinus. Normally, the medial wall fracture rarely extends above this horizontal line
- The entrapped orbital contents are reduced and the fracture segments of the medial wall are removed. This defines the whole boundary of medial wall defect. Titanium micromesh is used to cover this defect after trimming into an appropriate size
- Always recheck the position of implant after insertion as it may impinge upon medial rectus muscle

- Force duction test is performed to confirm proper placement of implant
- Wound is closed with 6-0 catgut sutures under microscope.

Endonasal Endoscopic Techniques

- ENT surgeons are well versed with this technique as they routinely do for Functional endoscopic surgeries (FESS)
- Usually performed under general anesthesia
- Decongestion is achieved with xylocaine 4% with adrenaline soaked cottonoids
- Uncinectomy followed by anterior ethmoidectomy with or without posterior ethmoidectomy is performed to complete the exposure
- The defect in lamina papyracea is visualized
- Fracture segments are removed and orbital contents are reduced
- Force duction test is performed to check any impingement of medial orbital muscle
- Nasal merocel pack is placed between the lamina papyracea defect and middle turbinate.

Advantages of Endoscopic Approaches

- No external scar
- Better access to posterior and superior orbital wall which is a constraint in other approaches
- Less duration of hospital stay.

Disadvantages

- Skilled expertise required
- Expensive endoscopic setup
- Chances of injury to lacrimal sac
- Increased chances of injury to lateral rectus muscle
- Intraoperative complications like cerebrospinal fluid (CSF) leak, optic nerve injury and epistaxis, etc.
- More chances of bone graft displacement with transcaruncular approach

Approach to Lateral Orbital Wall

Approach will be either through:

1. Extended subcilliary approach
2. Coronal approach.

Extended subciliary approach is used if there is isolated orbital wall fracture while coronal approach is used if there are other associated fractures as well.

Approaches to Superior Orbital Wall

1. Brow incision
2. Upper lid blepharoplasty
3. Coronal approach.

Brow incision and upper eyelid blepharoplasty approaches are generally used for isolated fractures of supraorbital region while coronal approach is used for orbital fracture associated with pan facial trauma fractures.

10

CHAPTER

Approaches to Frontal Bone Fracture

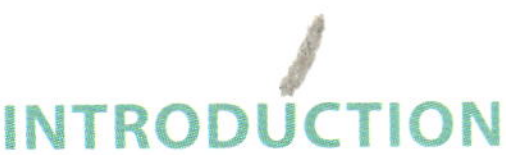

INTRODUCTION

Frontal bone fracture accounts for 5–15% of all maxillofacial injuries. The aim in treatment of fractures of frontal bone is to create a safe sinus that is to minimize the risk of potential complications related to injury. The complications which may arise are:

- Mucocele
- Mucopyocele
- Osteomyelitis
- Cerebral abscess.

These complications may not arise for many years following injury or repair. The fractures of frontal sinuses are divided into:

- Anterior wall fracture
- Posterior wall fracture
- Floor fracture
- Combination of these three fractures.

ANTERIOR WALL FRACTURE

Undisplaced anterior wall fractures are treated conservatively. Comminuted displaced fractures giving visual cosmetic deformity needs to be addressed. The various approaches are:

1. Open approach
   a. Brow incision
   b. Coronal incision.
2. Endoscopic approach.

Indications of Open Approaches

1. Done for comminuted anterior wall fractures causing esthetic defects.
2. Frontal sinus fracture associated other facial fractures.
3. Usually done for complex posterior frontal wall fracture associated with complications like cerebrospinal fluid (CSF) rhinorrhea, mucocele and exophthalmos.

Advantages

Gives good exposure.

Disadvantages

- Large visible scar
- Extensive dissection
- Alopecia
- Postoperative edema
- Paresthesia
- Injury to frontal branch of facial nerve.

BROW INCISION

Steps

Infiltration

Xylocaine 2% with adrenaline (1:2,00,000).

Incision

Incision is taken with 15 number blade through the skin parallel to superior border of eyebrow after marking with a surgical marker (Fig. 1).

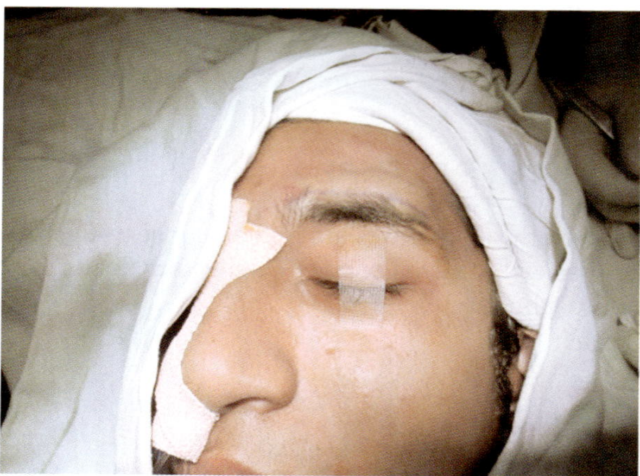

Fig. 1: Marking of brow incision

Dissection

- Dissection is continued through subcutaneous tissue and muscle layer (Fig. 2).

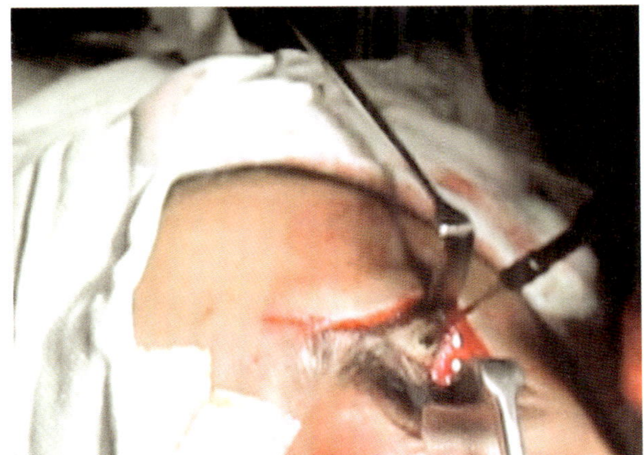

Fig. 2: Dissection through muscular layer

- Periosteum is sharply cut on reaching the anterior wall of the frontal bone (Fig. 3).

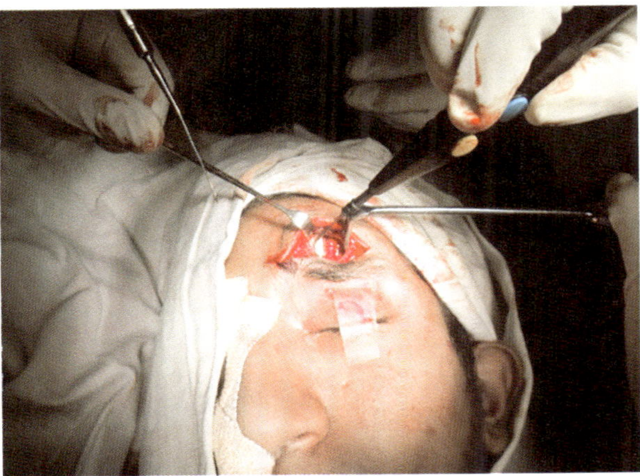

Fig. 3: Periosteum incision

- Utmost care should be taken to avoid any injury to supraorbital nerve (Fig. 4).

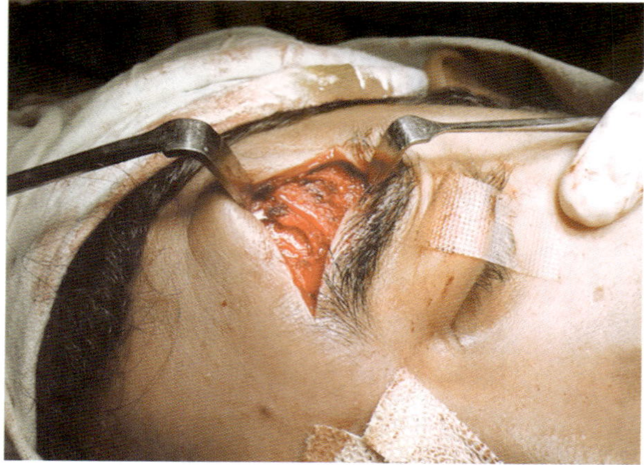

Fig. 4: Preservation of supraorbital nerve

- Appropriate reduction and fixation is done for the involved part of the frontal bone (Figs 5A and B).

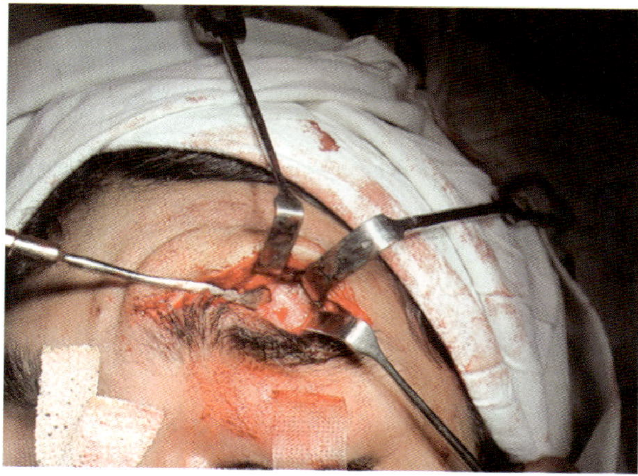

Fig. 5A: Reduction of the fracture segment

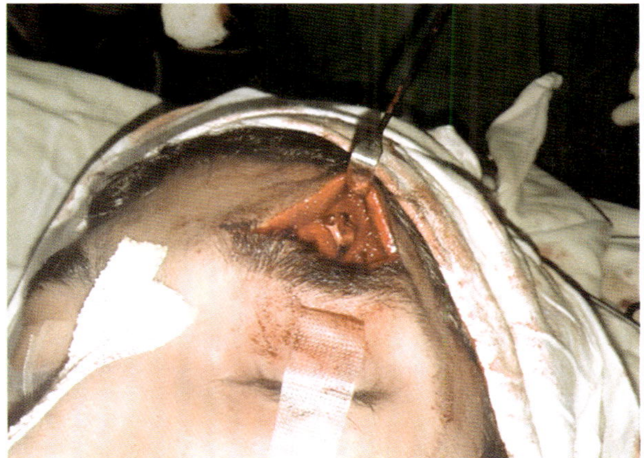

Fig. 5B: Exposure and fixation of fracture segment

Wound Closure (Fig. 6)

Closure is done in the following manner:

- Periosteum
- Muscle layer
- Skin.

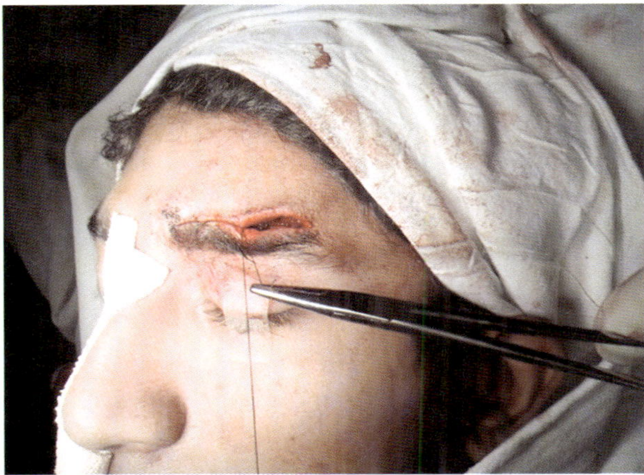

Fig. 6: Wound closure

Note: In case of placement of mesh at anterior wall through brow incision, sandwich technique can be used—in these technique, skin and muscle is dissected from down to up direction and then periosteum is incised and elevated from up to down direction—in such a way a pocket is created by periosteal flap in which mesh plate can be placed.

CORONAL INCISION

It is well described in Chapter 7 “Approaches to Zygomatic Fracture”.

ENDOSCOPIC APPROACHES

a. Intranasal
b. External.

Intranasal Endoscopic Approach

Indications

- To locate the frontal sinus ostium and plugging it:
  - Usually combined with open technique.

External Endoscopic Approach

Indications

- Generally used for isolated anterior table fracture which are limited to the vertical face of frontal bone)

(Injury with severe comminution and marked mucosal injuries of frontal sinus require open approach.)

- Isolated anterior table fracture is repaired for esthetic purpose only.

Techniques of External Endoscopic Technique

Preoperative considerations:

- Preoperative photograph of the defect
- Informed consent need to be taken for open approach in cases external endoscopic technique cannot be performed.

SURGICAL STEPS

- Patient head is painted and draped from orbit to vertex after endotracheal intubation
- Fracture line is marked and two incisions are taken

- One parasagittal incision (around 3–5 cm) is taken above from the fracture line. Working incision line is infiltrated with local agent. A stab incision is then taken over this line and a blind subperiosteal dissection is carried out till the fracture segment
- Another incision (around 1–2 cm) is taken at the same height of working incision line but 4–6 cm medial to it
- A scope is inserted through this incision and further dissection is carried out under scope guidance. Care must be taken to prevent injury to supratrochlear and supraorbital neurovascular bundle
- An implant of appropriate size and thickness is inserted through the working incision and brought to the fracture segment. This implant is stabilized by placement of screws. For insertion of the screws, a small incision is made at the exact site where implant has to be placed. A 1.7 mm self-drilling screw is passed through this incision and implant into the frontal bone thus securing the implant.

General Treatment of Frontal Sinus Fracture

1. Isolated anterior table fractures are repaired with reduced bony fragments attached to titanium mesh or by implants (isolated anterior table fracture are normally managed conservatively and needs to be addressed only for cosmetic defect) .
2. Isolated anterior table fractures which are old enough and cannot be reduced, can be camouflaged with bone cement or vascularized calvarial graft.
3. Anterior table fractures with nasofrontal duct involvement are repaired by sinus obliteration and anterior wall reconstruction with reduced bony fragments attached to titanium mesh or implant.
4. Anterior and posterior table fractures with cerebrospinal fluid leak or displacement are treated with the cranialization of the sinus and anterior wall reconstruction with reduced bony fragments attached to titanium mesh.

Bone Graft Harvesting

BONE GRAFTS

Primary Bone Graft

They are commonly used to restore the integrity of:

- Orbital wall
- Mid facial buttress
- Nose
- Frontal bone area
- Mandible

The commonly harvested grafts in clinical practice are:

1. Iliac crest
2. Calvarial graft
3. Rib graft

Bone grafts are used to maintain facial height and projection. They are also harvested for filling structural defects. It augments and hastens the healing potential and strength of bone consolidation.

Contraindications

- Infected/Contaminated wound
- Gunshot wound where the critical areas of soft tissue are missing.

ILIAC CREST

Advantages

- It is one of the most common donor sites
- It can be easily moulded to give required shape
- Large segments of cortical, cancellous or corticocancellous bone can be quickly harvested for varying size defects

- The location of the ilium allows harvesting by a different surgical team to save operative duration
- A full-thickness iliac graft would have two thick cortices with plenty of trabecular bone which resembles closely to the height and thickness of the mandible.

Disadvantages

- High chances of absorption
- Postoperative pain and limping.

Anterior Iliac Grafts

Large amount of cancellous or corticocancellous segments can be obtained from the anterior ilium.

Steps

- Incise with a cautery knife along the iliac crest, avoiding muscle. Subperiosteally, dissect the abdominal musculature and, subsequently, the iliacus from the inner wall of the ilium (Fig. 1)

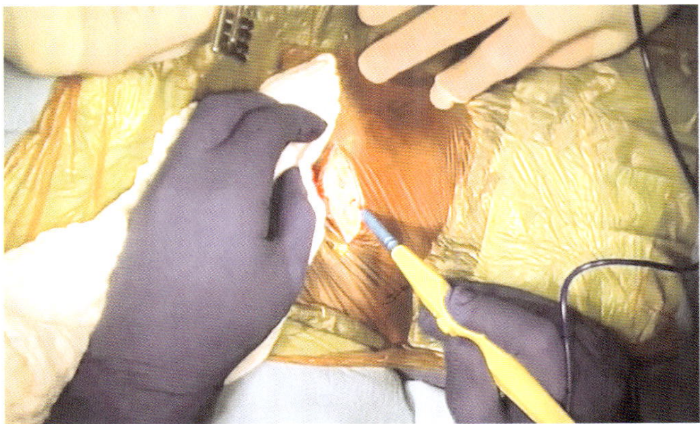

Fig. 1: Making of incision along the iliac crest

- Outline the area to be harvested with the help of osteotomes. Cut the required amount of bony strips (Fig. 2)
- Harvest the corticocancellous strips with a gouge and remove additional cancellous bone with gouges and curets (Fig. 3).

Posterior Iliac Grafts

The region of the posterosuperior iliac spine is the best source of cancellous bone.

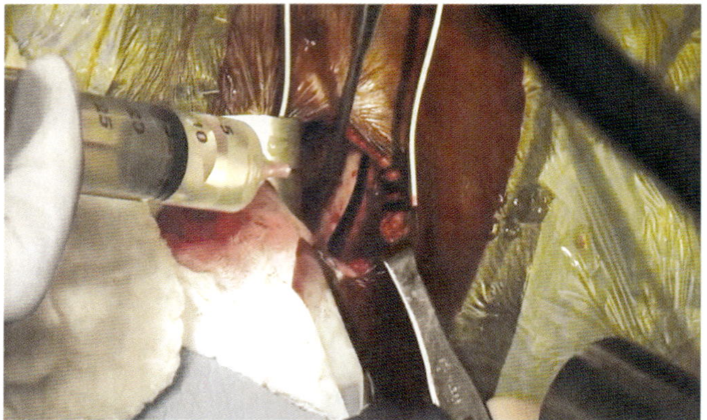

Fig. 2: Stripping of bony graft

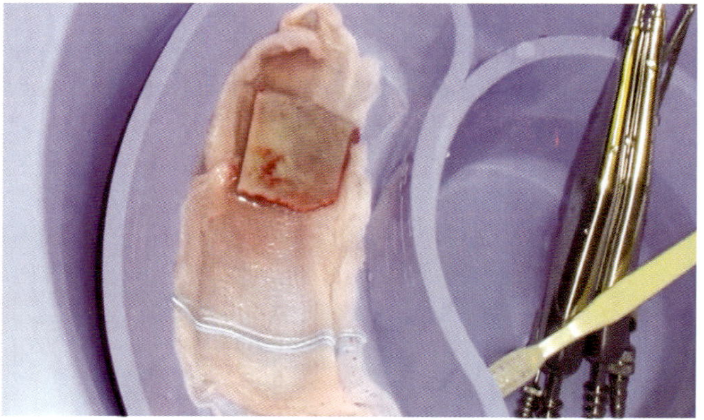

Fig. 3: Harvested piece of bone graft

Complications

- Postoperative pain
- Unsightly contour defects along the iliac crest
- Acetabular or iliac fractures or instability
- Neurovascular injury.

CALVARIAL GRAFT

This is one of the most popular cortical bone grafts in craniofacial reconstruction, mainly for its mechanical properties and very slow resorption rate. This makes it ideal for facial augmentation and covering cranial defects.

Advantages

- It can be harvested with bicoronal flaps
- Large area can be harvested
- Full thickness or split thickness can be used.

Disadvantages

- Avascular, brittle and difficult to shape and contour
- Chances of neurological complications
- Chances of dural tear
- Chances of hemotoma.

There are several key anatomic facts to consider before harvesting a calvarial bone graft:

- Thickness of the calvarium is highly variable
- The dura is firmly adherent to the inner cortex and can be easily injured if the inner cortex is to be harvested with the graft
- Various important vascular structures lies immediately beneath the inner cortex
- Other anatomic variables, including transcortical emissary veins, subcortical vessels, and aberrant arachnoid plexuses, should also be considered
- The temporoparietal region provides more curved bone, which would be more suitable for orbital or malar reconstruction. However, straight grafts can be harvested more posteriorly (i.e. from the occipitoparietal region). Generally, the bone is harvested as narrow strips to avoid graft fracture during harvest and then, several strips can be fixed together and used as one graft.

Calvarial Bone can be Harvested at Three Levels

1. Partial-thickness outer cortex
2. Full-thickness outer cortex
3. Bicortical
   - Partial-thickness outer cortex can be harvested using a very sharp osteotome to shave off a sheet of cortical bone
   - In adults, full-thickness outer cortex can safely be harvested and is, therefore, the most commonly used calvarial graft
   - If a craniotomy has already been performed, the inner cortex can be harvested from the bone flap and used in the reconstruction, leaving the outer cortex to be placed back in its original position. This technique maintains the contour of the calvarium
   - If large quantities of bone are needed, bicortical grafts may be harvested, followed by splitting of the two cortices to double the surface area of the graft (Figs 4A and B).

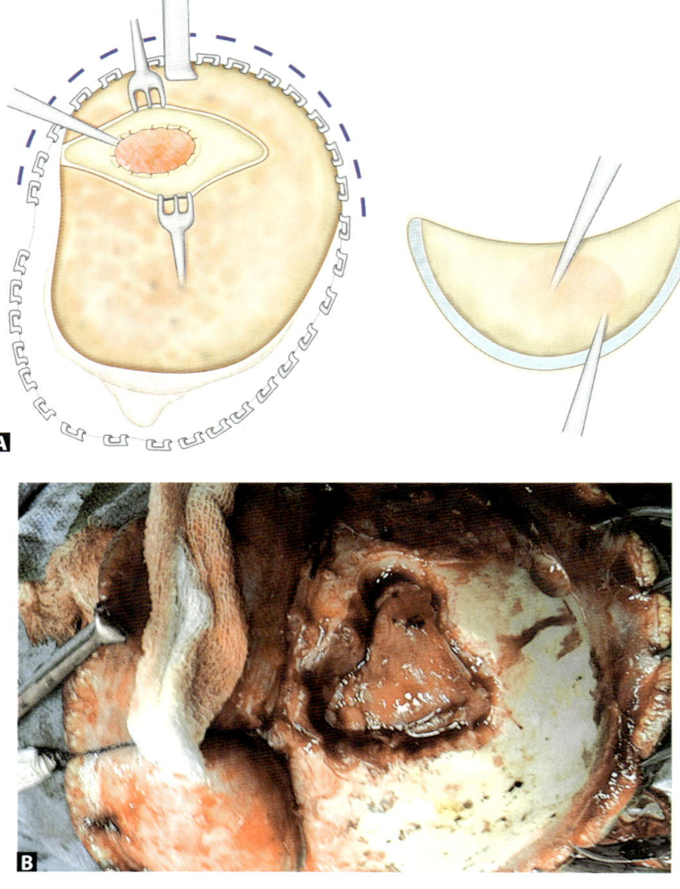

Figs 4A and B: Bicoronal flap with defect left over after calvarial graft

Complications of Calvarial Graft

- Surface deformity at the donor and/or recipient site
- Chances of graft fracture during harvest
- Dural exposure or tear (if the dura is injured, it should be patched either with a temporalis fascia or, more recently, a synthetic graft)
- Rarely intracranial hemorrhage.

RIB GRAFT

- Nonvascularized rib was the first autogenous bone graft used for reconstruction of mandibular segmental defects

- Osseous or osseochondral segments can be harvested from ribs 5 to 7 and can be used either in full or in split thickness
- Costochondral grafts are very popular in the treatment of ramus and condylar defects
- Commonly used for augmentation rhinoplasty.

Advantages

- It can be used as a full or split thickness graft
- Easy to contour in various shapes
- Marrow can be curetted out of the split rib to provide a smooth contour
- Multiple ribs can be harvested in cases of large defect.

Disadvantages

- Chances of injury to neurovascular bundle
- Postoperative pain which may require potent analgesics
- Chances of pleural tear.

Steps

- Dissection through the latissimus dorsi and trapezius muscles exposes the rib and facilitates harvest (Figs 5A and B).

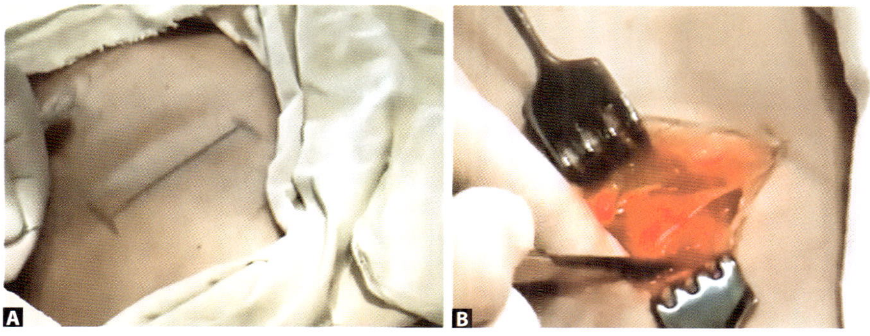

Figs 5A and B: (A) Marking of incision; (B) Dissection to expose the rib

- The periosteum over the rib is incised, either with the use of electrocautery or sharply with a scalpel, and a periosteal elevator is used to strip the superficial portion of the rib (Fig. 6)
- A rib stripper is then used subperiosteally to completely strip the pleural surface of the rib. This maneuver is performed all the way to the vertebral and sternal ends of the ribs (Fig. 7)

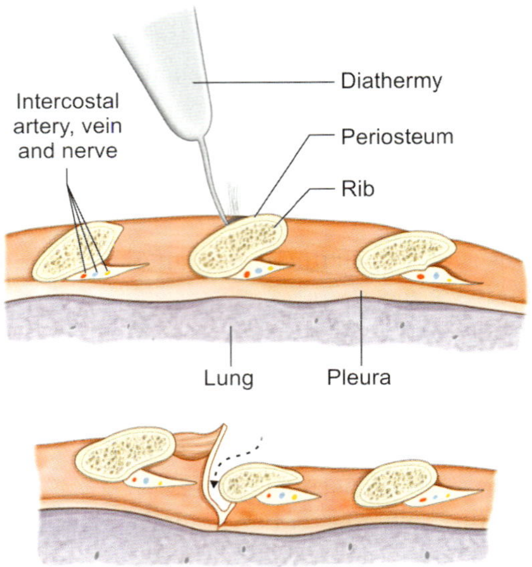

Fig. 6: Showing schematic picture of harvesting of rib graft

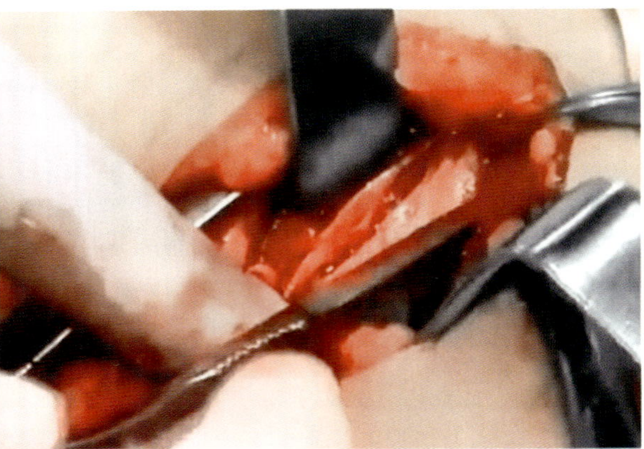

Fig. 7: Showing use of periosteum elevator to completely strip off the rib

- A rib cutter is then used to excise the required amount of graft (Figs 8 and 9).

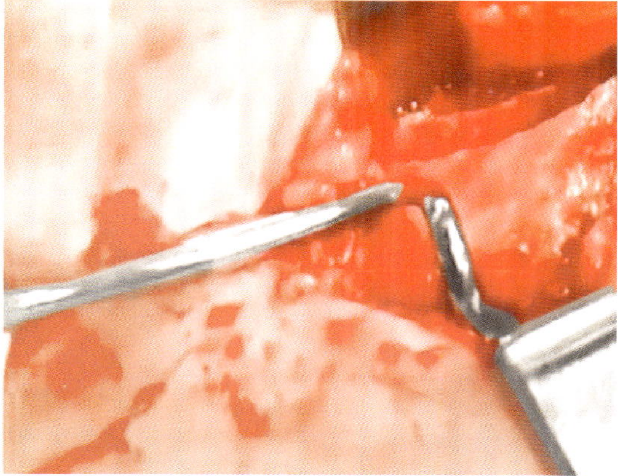

Fig. 8: Use of rib shear to obtain the graft

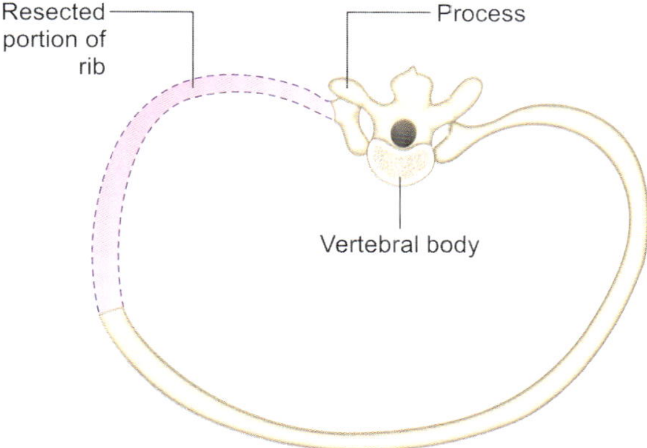

Fig. 9: Schematic picture of area which can be resected to obtain rib graft

Side Effects and Complications

- Postoperative chest-wall pain
- Pleural injury leading to pneumothorax or pleuritis.

SURGICAL ATLAS

CASE 1: SYMPHYSIS FRACTURE (INTRAORAL APPROACH)

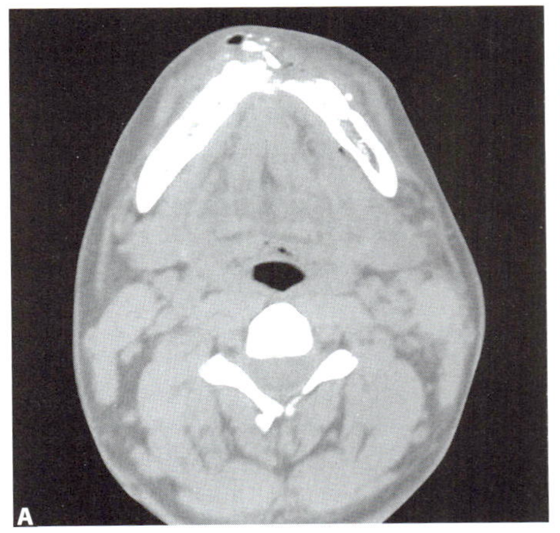

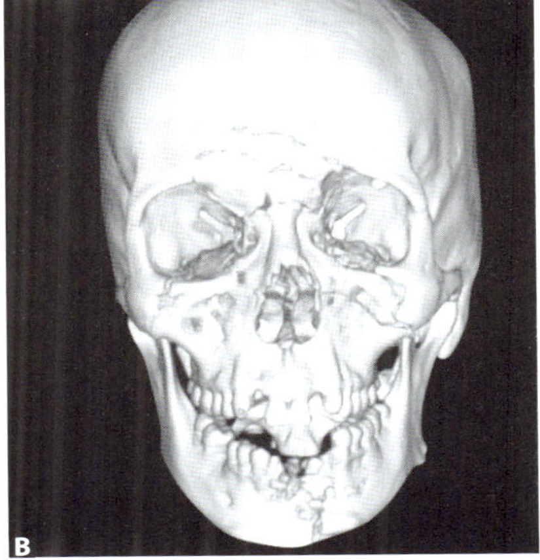

Figs 1A and B: CT scan showing fracture line passing through the symphysis region

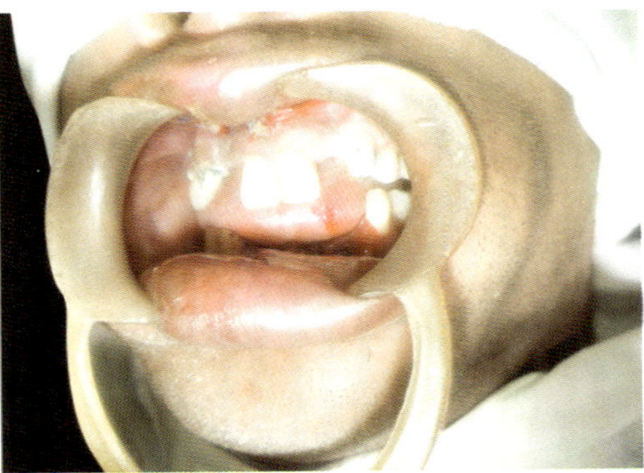

Fig. 2: Preoperative occlusion (missing tooth and posterior open bite)

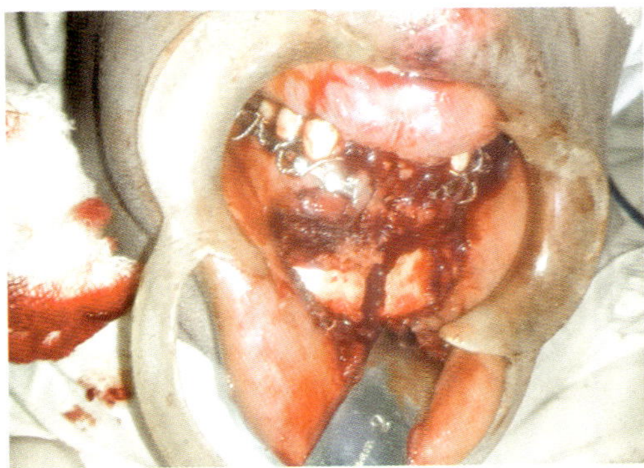

Fig. 3: Intraoperative picture showing the fracture site

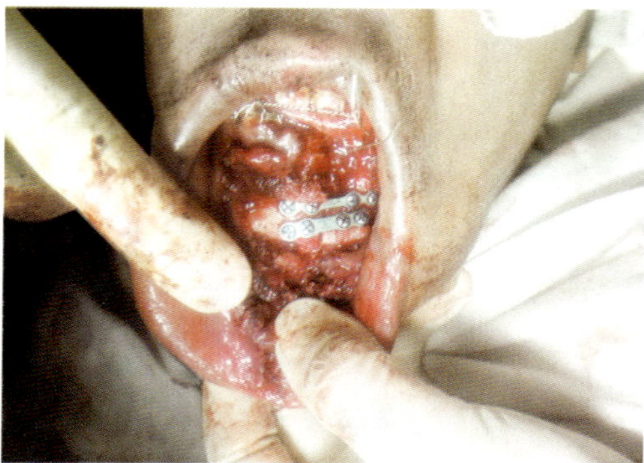

Fig. 4: Intraoperative picture showing open reduction and internal fixation of the fracture site with 4 hole plates (with gap) with 2 holes on either sides of the fracture line; one plate at the upper border and another one at the lower border of the mandible

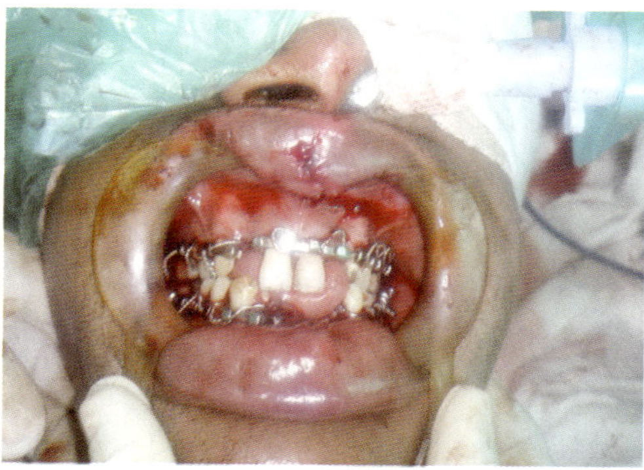

Fig. 5: Postoperative occlusion after the reduction and internal fixation

CASE 2: PARASYMPHYSIS FRACTURE (INTRAORAL APPROACH)

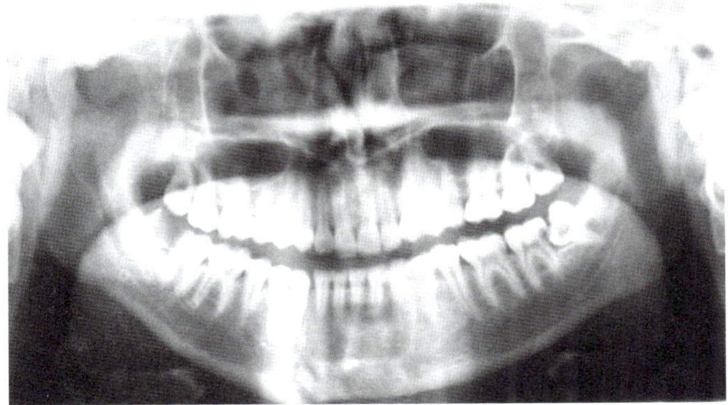

Fig. 6: Orthopantomogram (OPG) showing fracture line passing through right side parasymphysis region

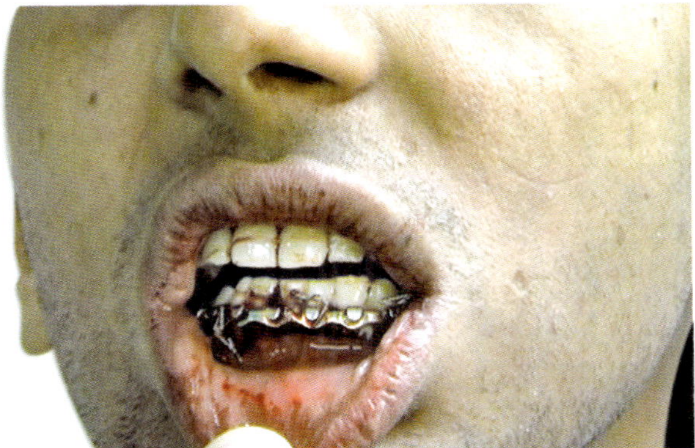

Fig. 7: Preoperative picture of the patient showing malocclusion

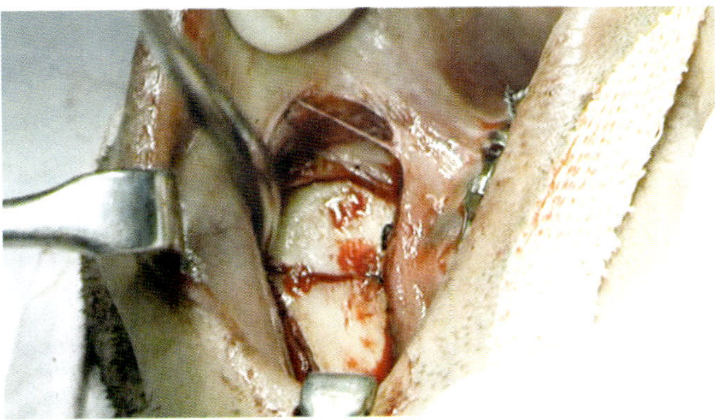

Fig. 8: Intraoral approach to expose the fracture site

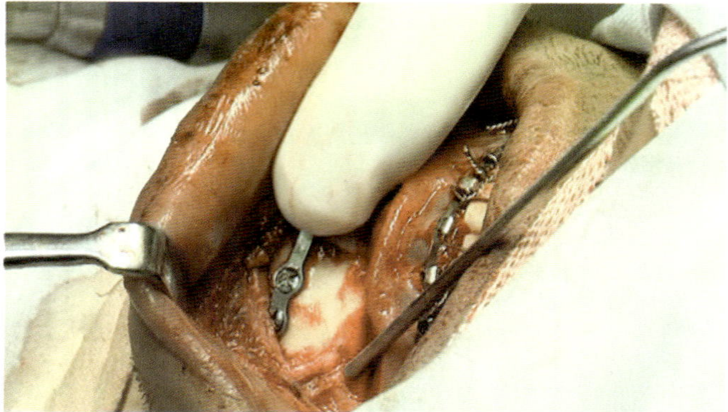

Fig. 9: Internal fixation with 4 hole miniplate with 2 holes on either sides of the fracture line with secured mental nerve and vessels

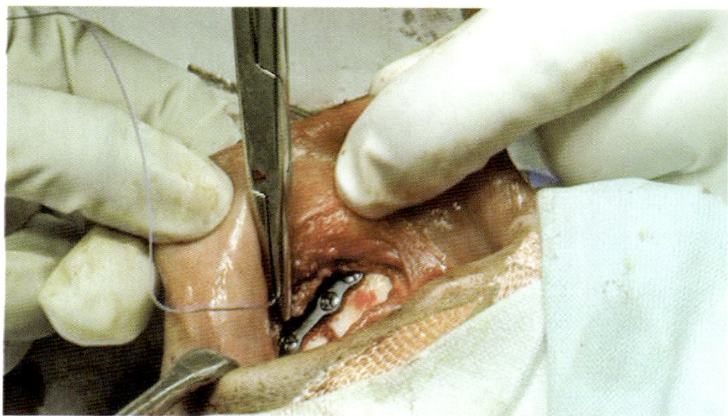

Fig. 10: Closure of the wound in layers

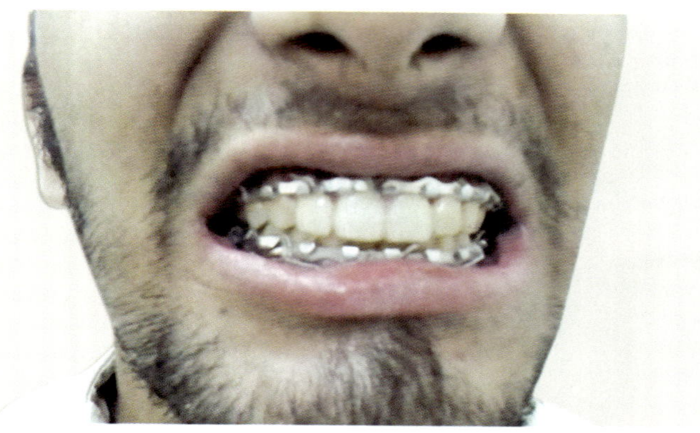

Fig. 11: Postoperative normal occlusion

CASE 3: BODY MANDIBLE

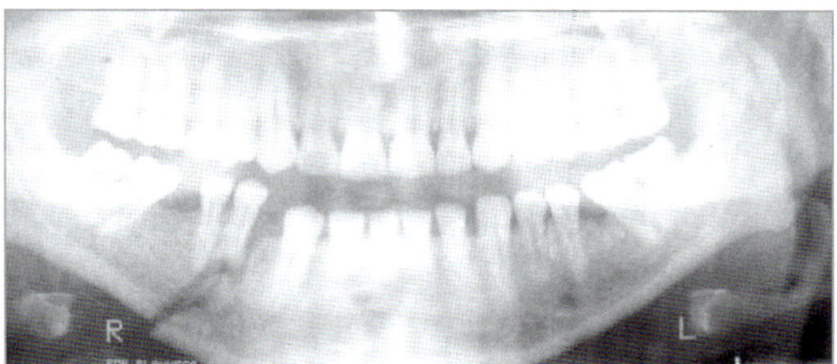

Fig. 12: Orthopantomogram showing fracture line passing through body of mandible on the right side

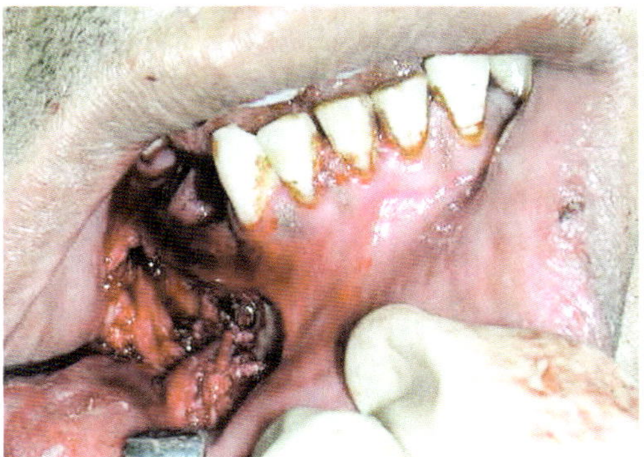

Fig. 13: Open reduction and internal fixation with mini-hole plates

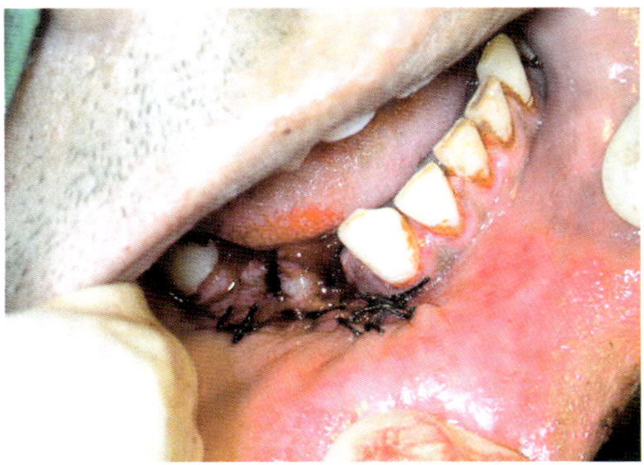

Fig. 14: Closure of the wound in layers

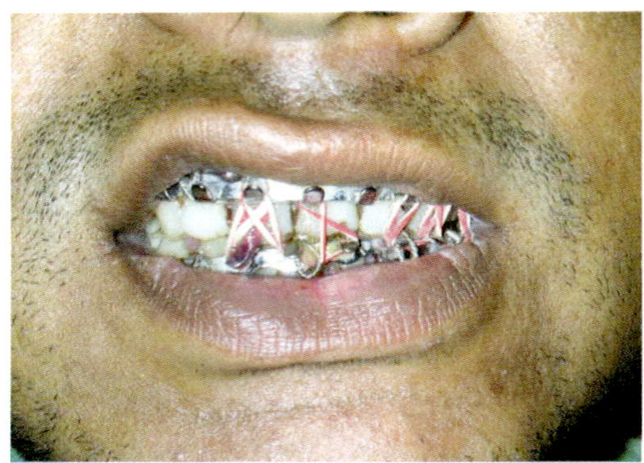

Fig. 15: Postoperative picture showing normal occlusion and securing the intermaxillary fixation with elastic bands

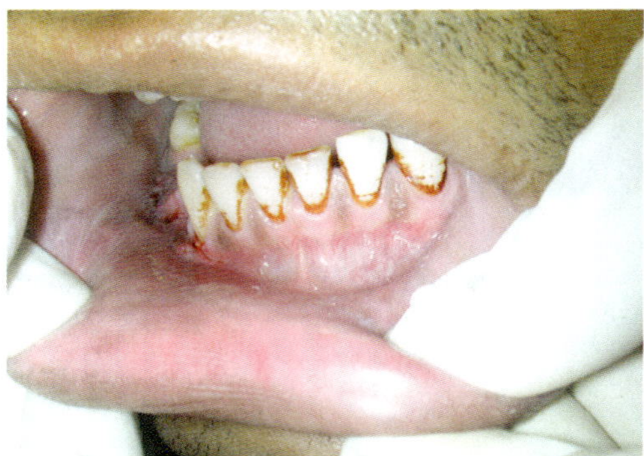

Fig. 16: Postoperative 10th day picture showing healed scar with maintained gingivobuccal sulcus

CASE 4: ANGLE MANDIBLE

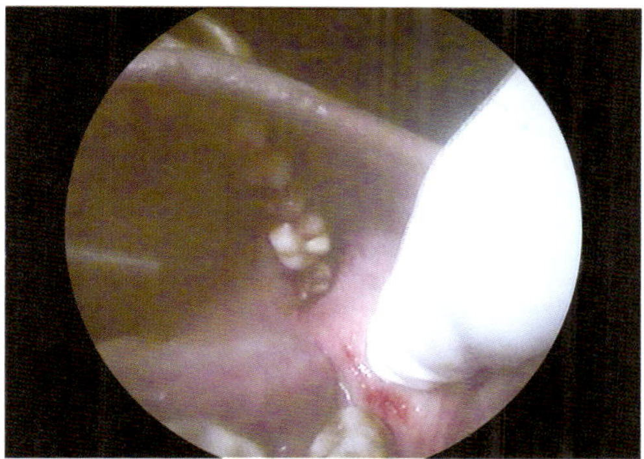

Fig. 17: Incision line over the fracture site (0.5 cm away from attached margin of the gingiva)

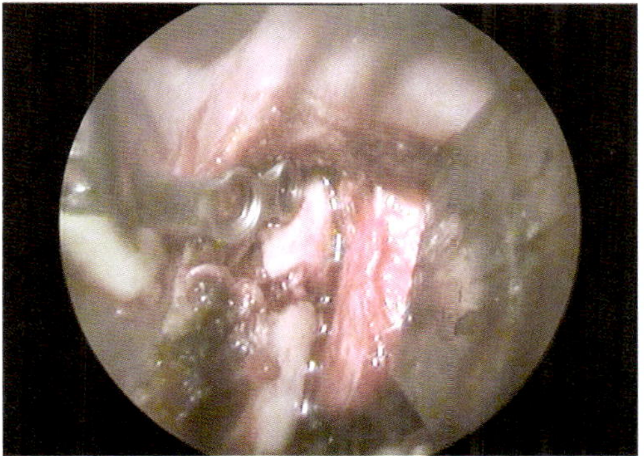

Fig. 18: Exposure of the fracture site

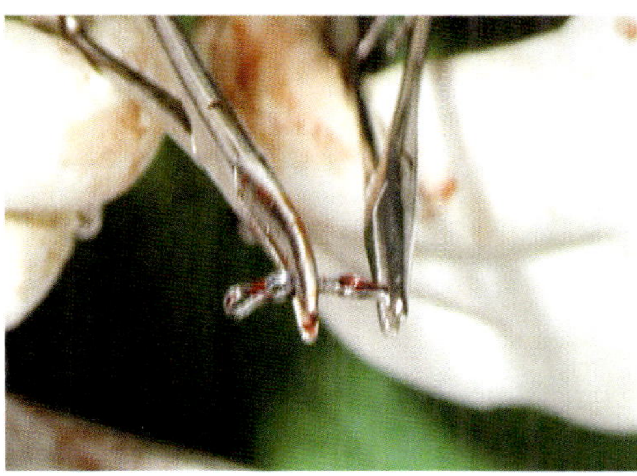

Fig. 19: Adapting the plate by rotating one end of the mini-plate by 90°

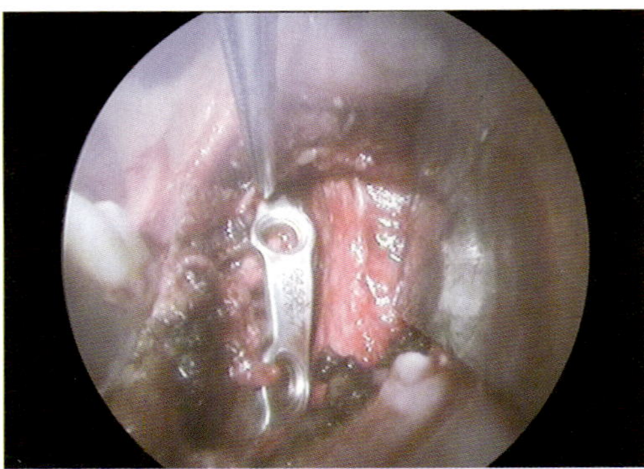

Fig. 20: Adapted plate placed over the fracture site in such a way that 2 holes of the mini-plate lies over either side of fracture line

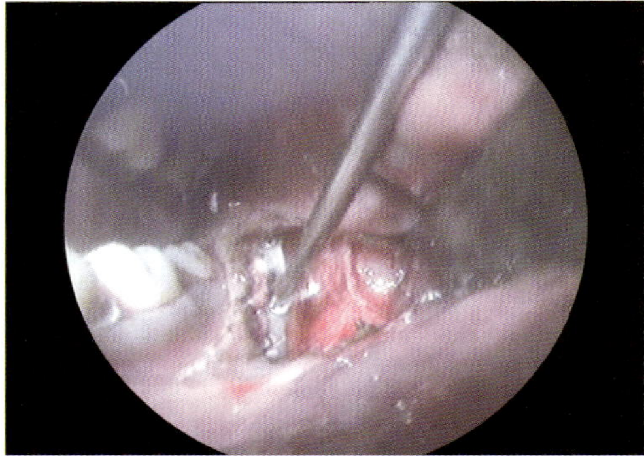

Fig. 21: Securing the plate with appropriate screws

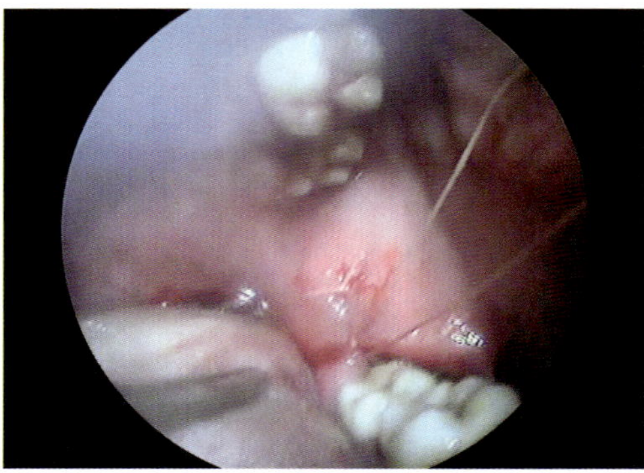

Fig. 22: Closure of the wound in layers

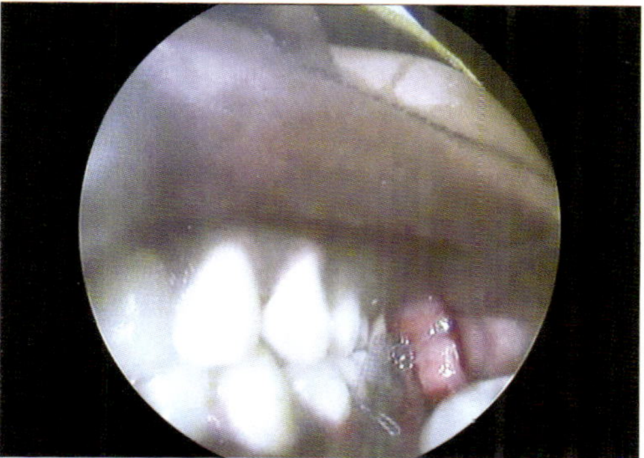

Fig. 23: Postoperative picture showing r ormal occlusion

CASE 5: SUBCONDYLAR FRACTURE (RETROMANDIBULAR APPROACH)

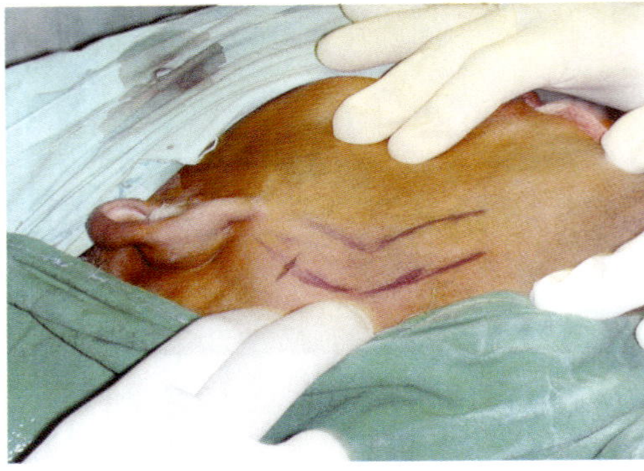

Fig. 24: Incision taken few millimeters away from posterior border of the mandible

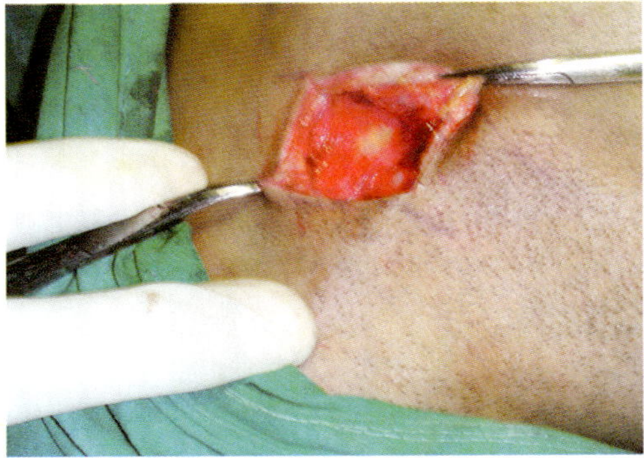

Fig. 25: Exposure of the pterygomandibular sling

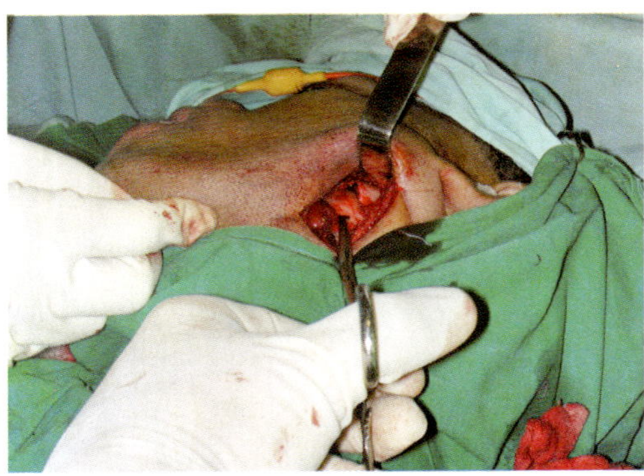

Fig. 26: Manipulation of the fracture segment to bring it in alignment

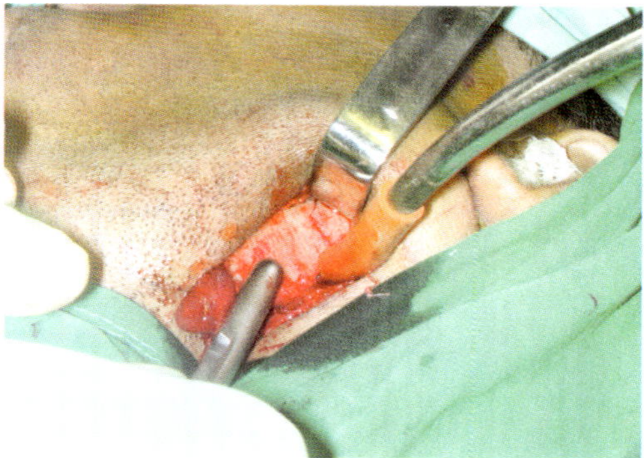

Fig. 27: Fracture segments after reduction

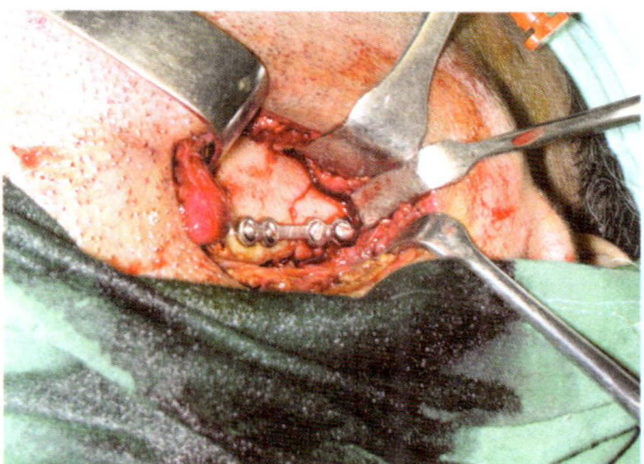

Fig. 28: Internal fixation with 4 hole mini-hole plate with 2 holes on either sides of fracture line

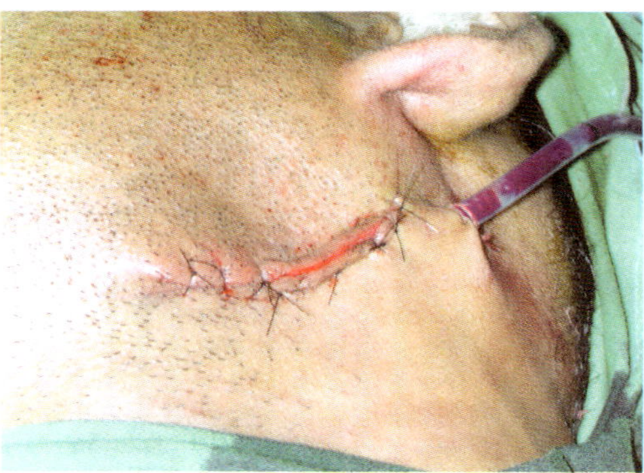

Fig. 29: Closure of wound in layers with drain in-situ

CASE 6: INFRAORBITAL FRACTURE (SUBCILIARY APPROACH)

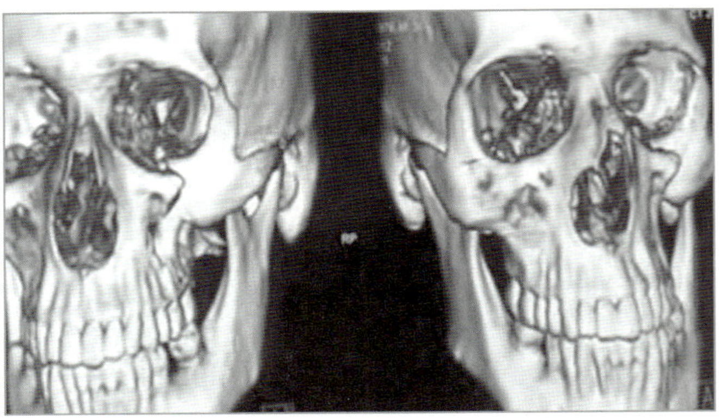

Fig. 30: 3D-CT scan showing infraorbital rim fracture on the left side

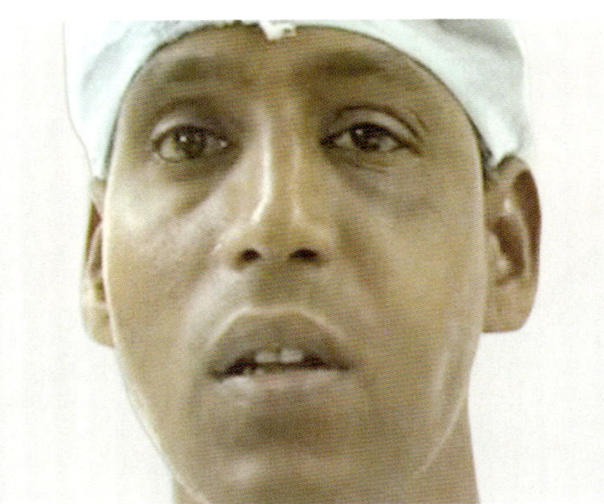

Fig. 31: Preoperative picture of the patient showing depression over infraorbital region on the left side

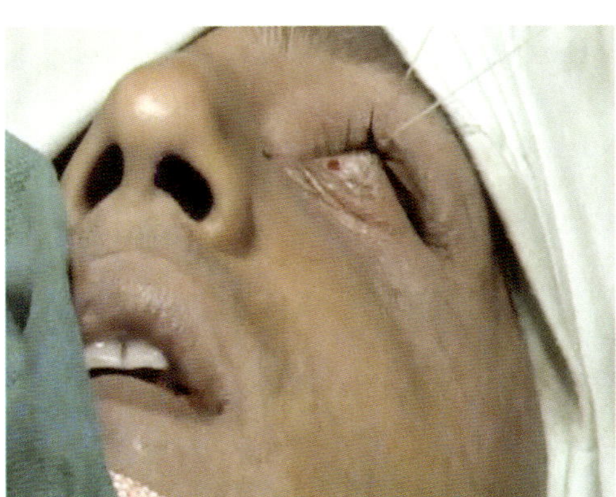

Fig. 32: Temporary tarsorrhaphy to protect the eyeball

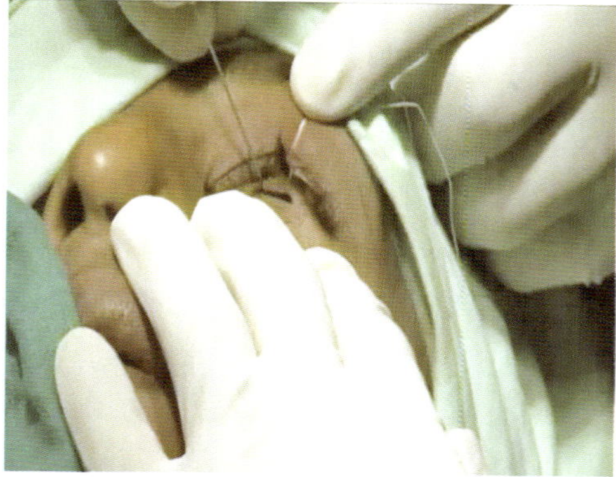

Fig. 33: Marking for the subciliary incision

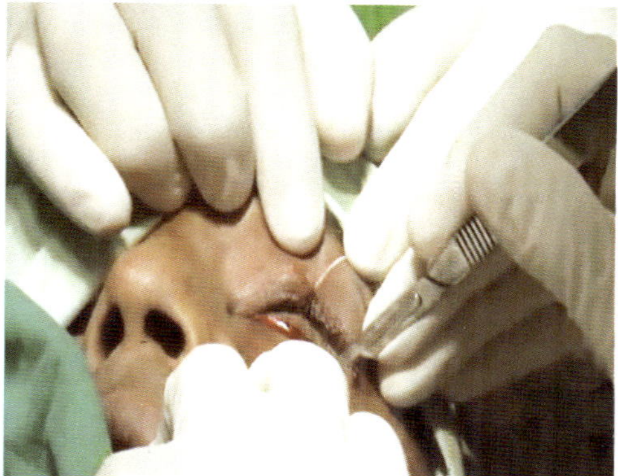

Fig. 34: Subciliary incision taken few millimeters away from the lower eye lashes

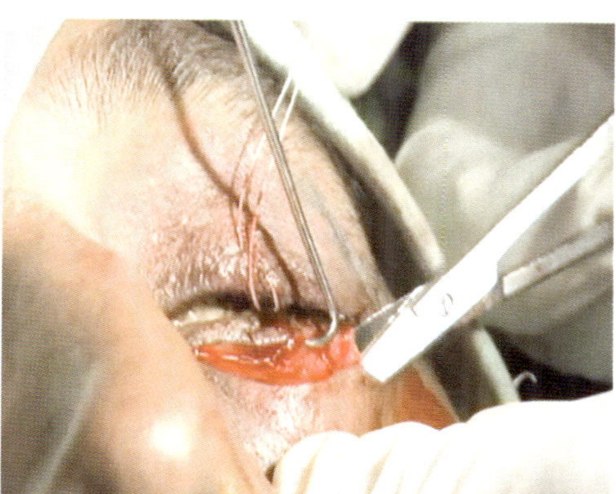

Fig. 35: Orbicularis occularis muscle cut to obtain the plane between muscle and the orbital septa

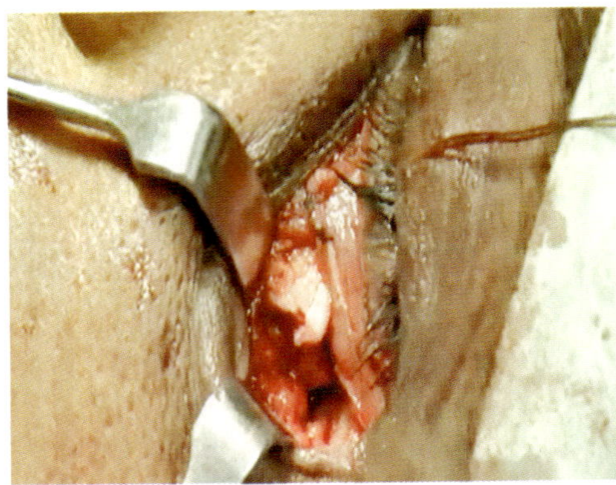

Fig. 36: Fracture site well exposed

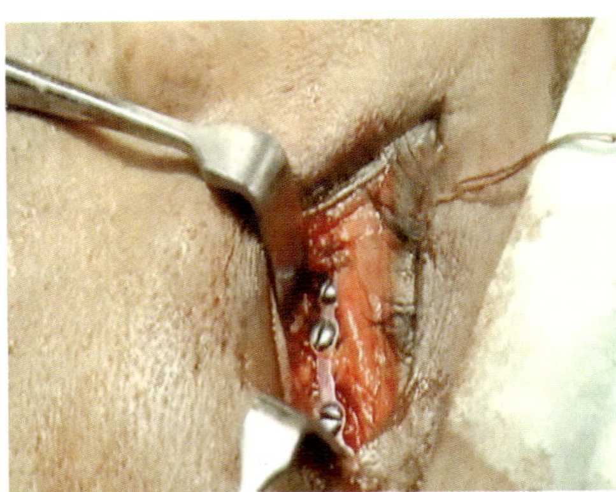

Fig. 37: Reduction with internal fixation of the fracture segments with mini-hole plate

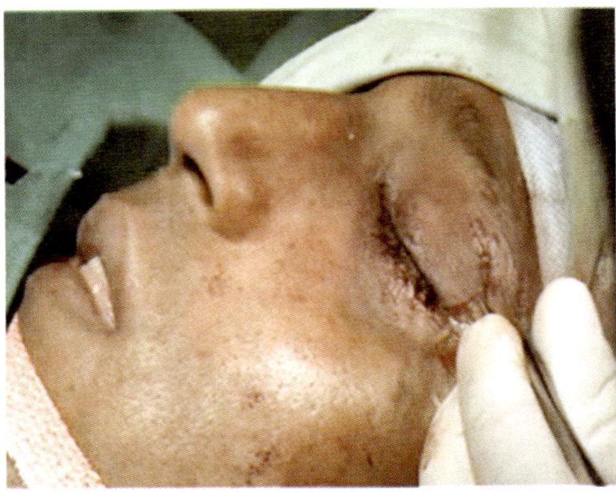

Fig. 38: Immediate postoperative picture with closed surgical wound and normal facial symmetry

CASE 7: THREE POINT FIXATION USING EXISTING WOUND (TRIPOD FRACTURE)

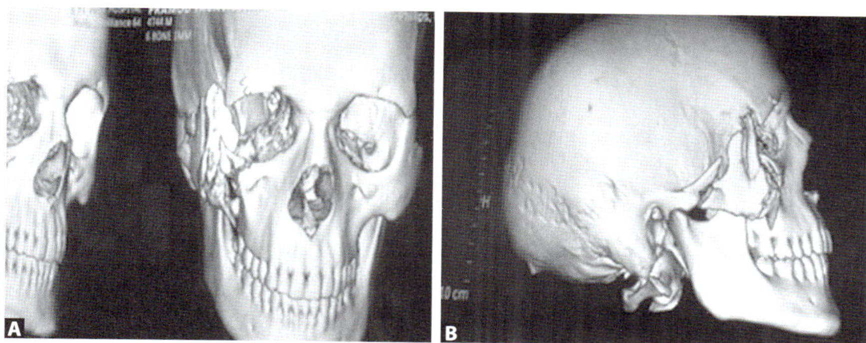

Figs 39A and B: CT Scan showing communited fractures involving infraorbital rim, zygomaticomaxillary buttress and zygomaticofrontal suture and body of zygoma

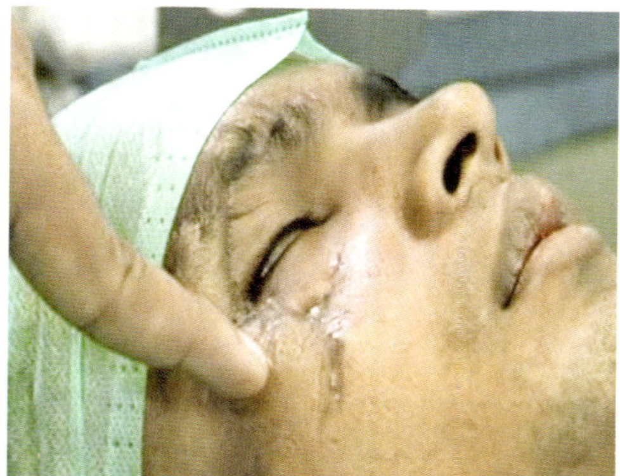

Fig. 40: Preoperative picture showing healed scar over fracture site with cosmetic deformity

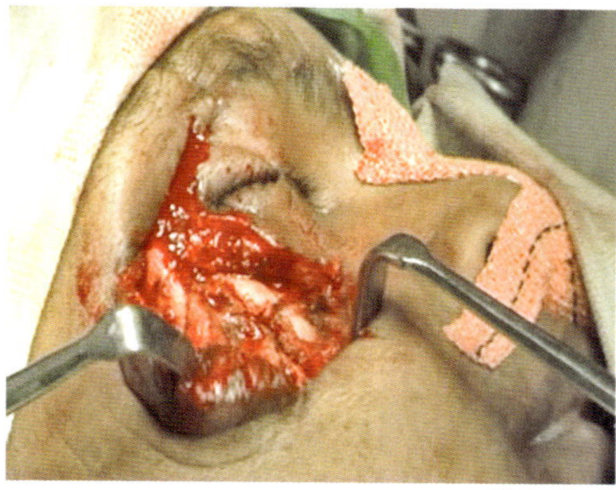

Fig. 41: Extrapolation of existing scar to expose the fracture site

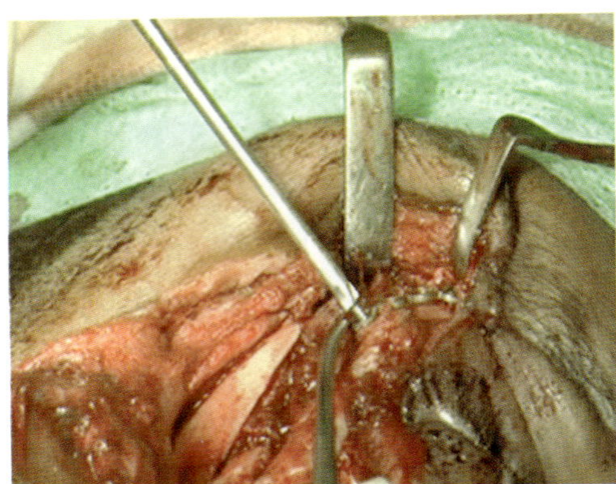

Fig. 42: Fixation of zygomaticofrontal suture line with part of reconstruction plate

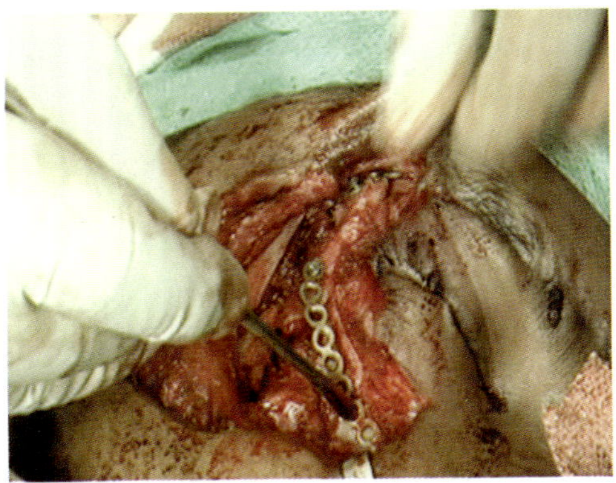

Fig. 43: Fixation of infraorbital rim fracture with reconstruction plate

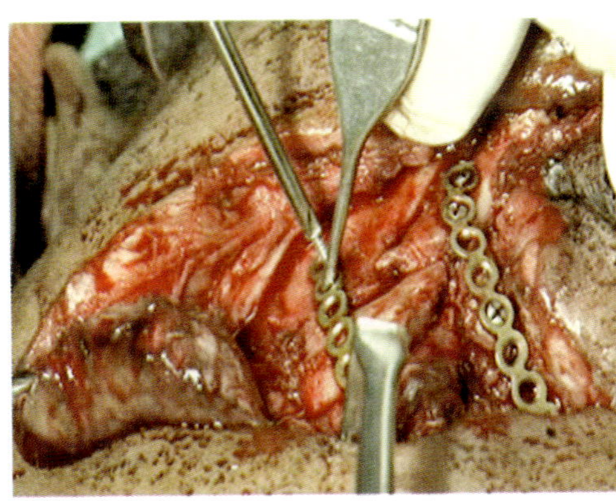

Fig. 44: Fixation of zygomaticomaxillary buttress with part of reconstruction plate

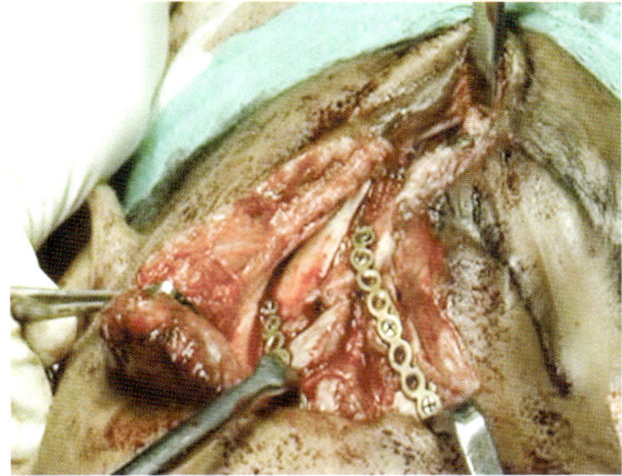

Fig. 45: Three point fixation achieved with ORIF

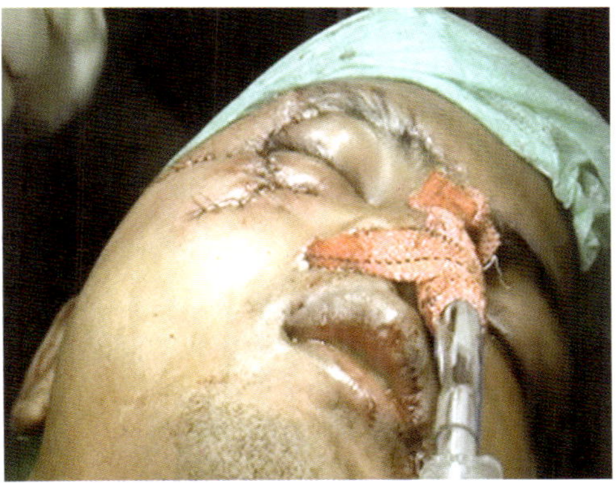

Fig. 46: Immediate postoperative picture showing revised suturing of the wound with normal facial symmetry

CASE 8: FRONTAL FRACTURE (SUPRAORBITAL APPROACH)

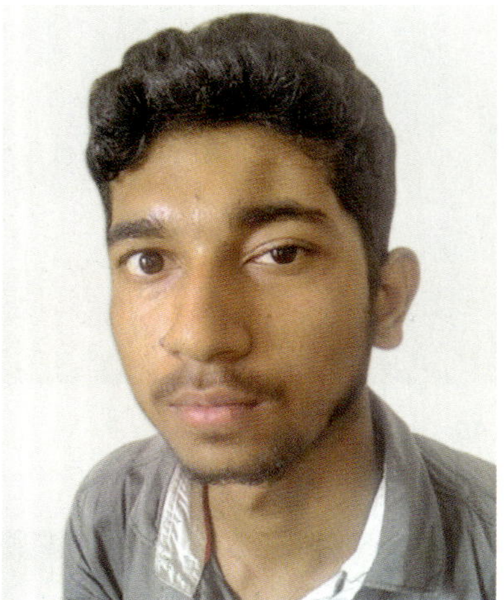

Fig. 47: Post-traumatic cosmetic deformity over frontal region on the left side

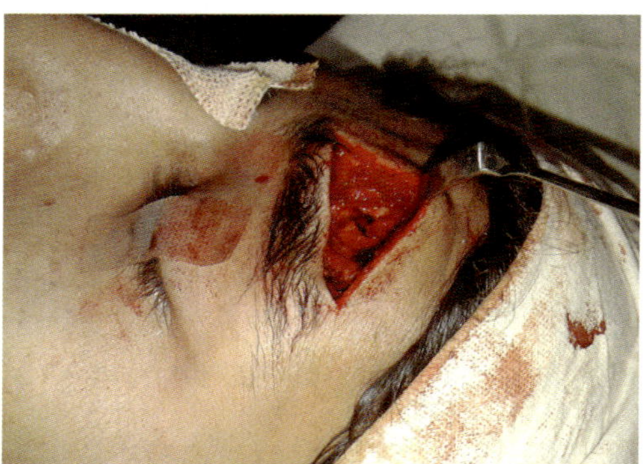

Fig. 48: Supraorbital approach to expose the fracture site

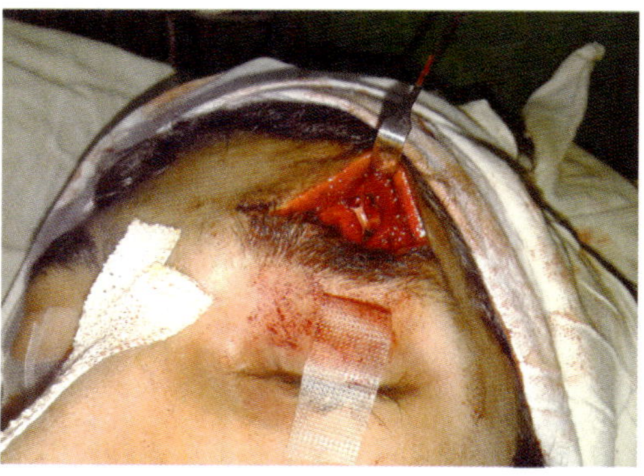

Fig. 49: Open reduction and internal fixation with mini-hole plates

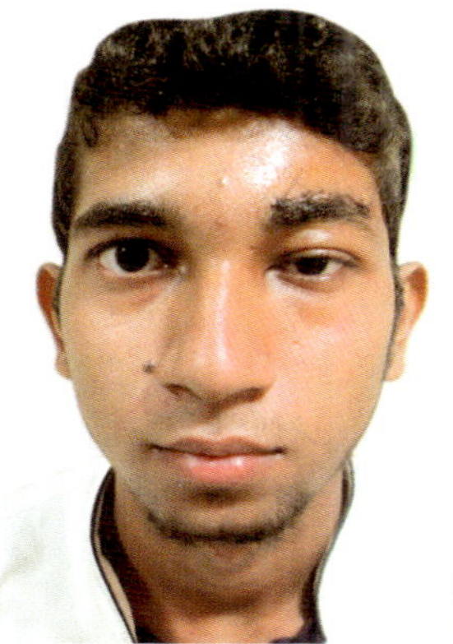

Fig. 50: Postoperative 7th day picture showing normal facial symmetry

CASE 9: FRONTAL MUCOCELE

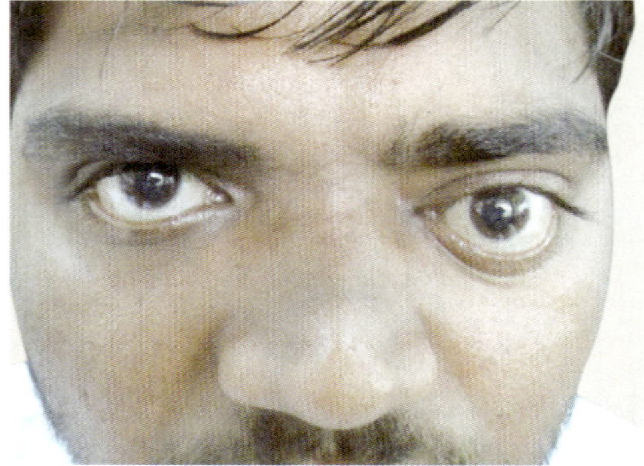

Fig. 51: Preoperative picture of a patient with marked proptosis following orbital roof fracture having preexisting frontal mucocele

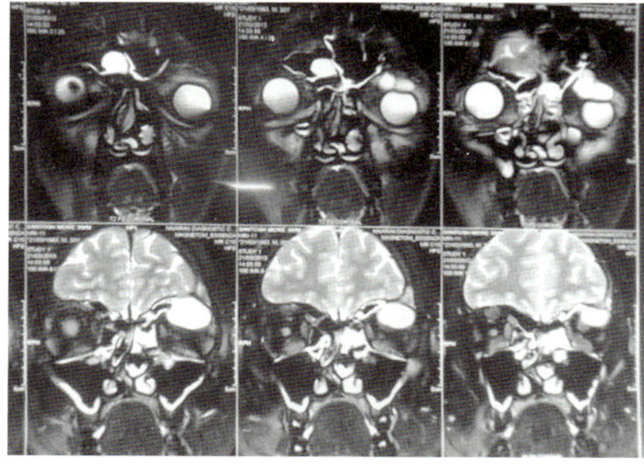

Fig. 52: MR scan showing mucocele compressing the eyeball on the left side

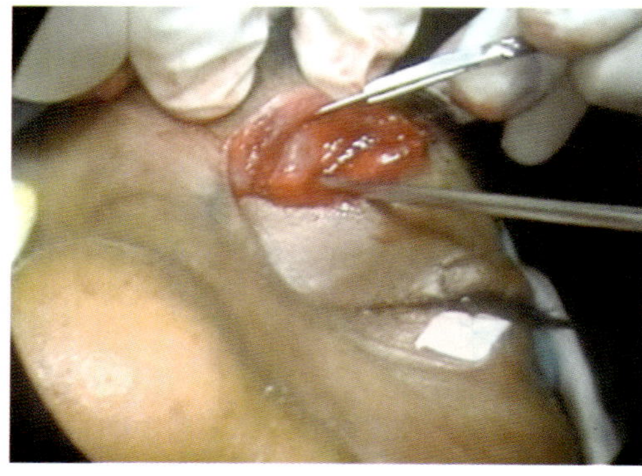

Fig. 53: Brow incision taken to access the orbital roof

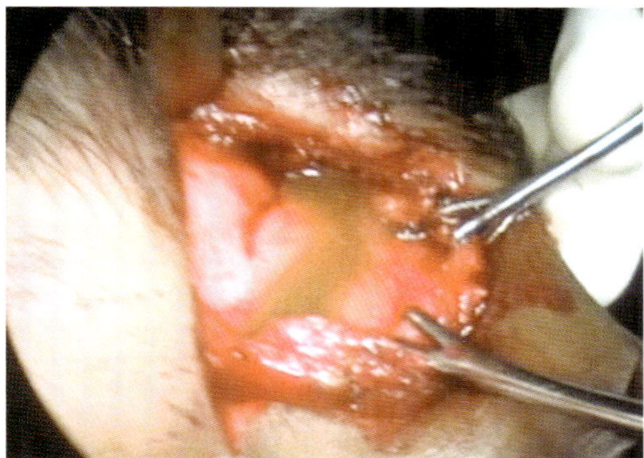

Fig. 54: Fluid coming out of the ruptured mucocele

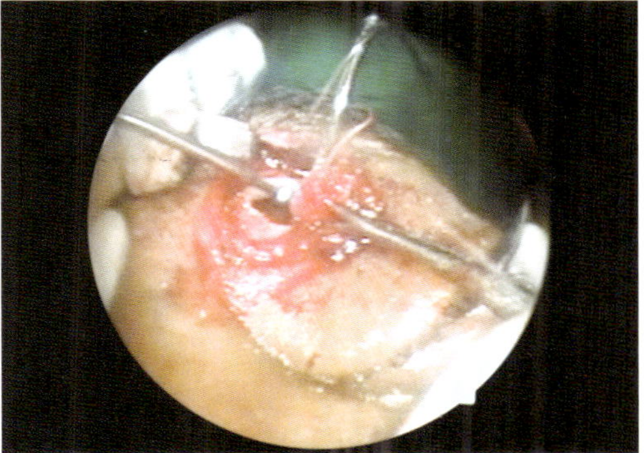

Fig. 55: Drilling the anterior table of the frontal sinus to access the sinus cavity

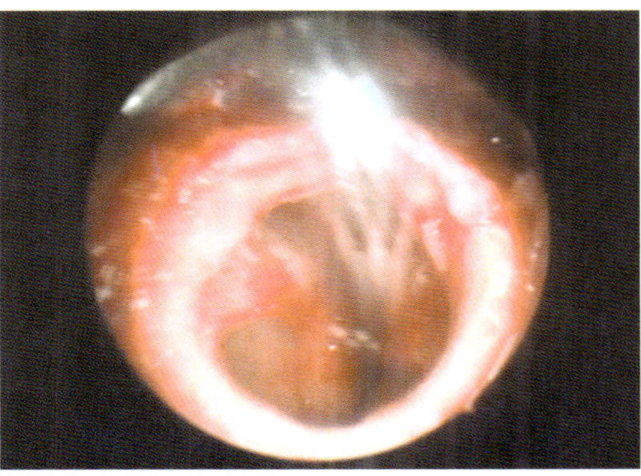

Fig. 56: Complete denudation of the sinus off its mucosa (which was later obliterated with muscle and fat)

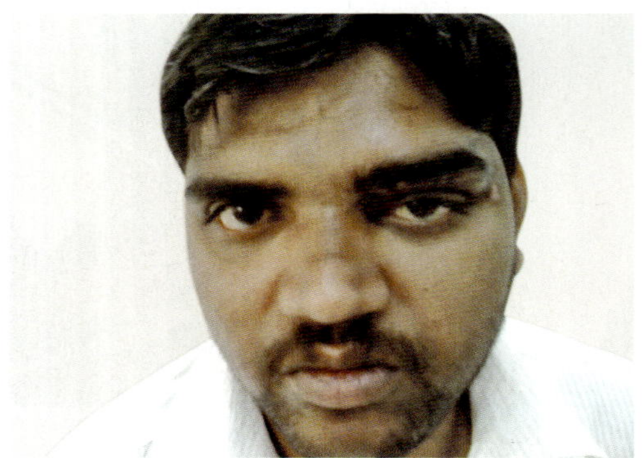

Fig. 57: Postoperative picture of the patient with inconspicuous scar and normal eyeball

CASE 10: TEMPOROMANDIBULAR JOINT ARTHOPLASTY

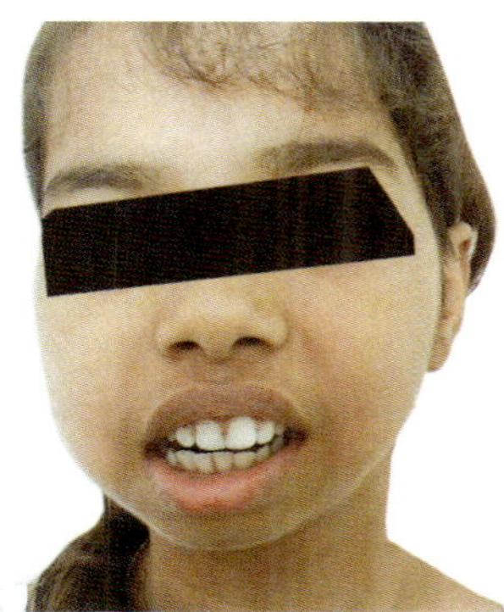

Fig. 58: Preoperative picture of the patient having temporomandibular joint ankylosis following post-traumatic subconcylar fracture

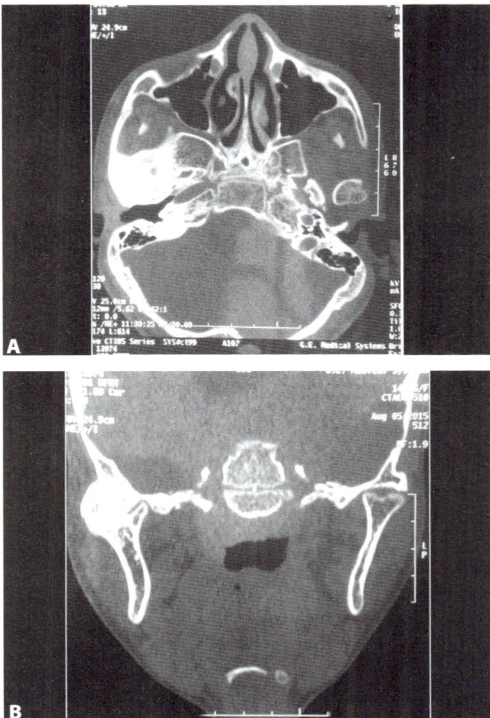

Figs 59A and B: CT images showing fused right side mandibular condyle with skull base

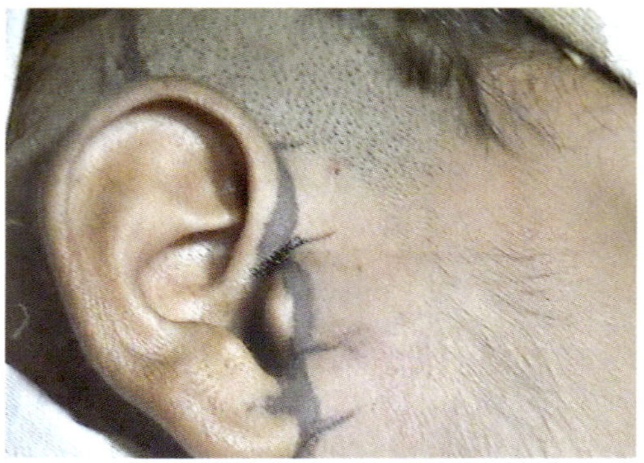

Fig. 60: Modified preauricular incision (Alkayat- Bramley incision)

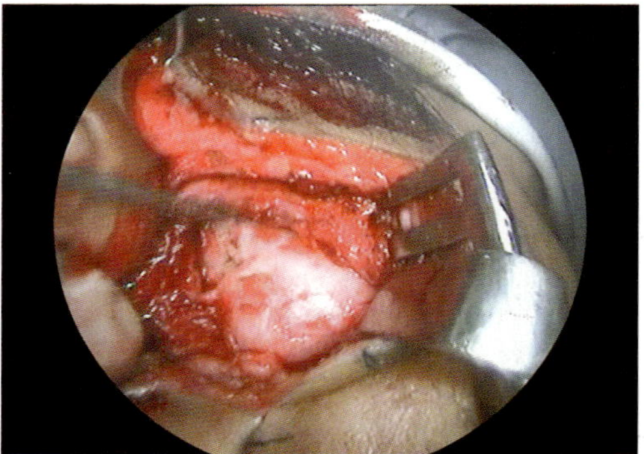

Fig. 61: Exposure of ankylosed TM joint

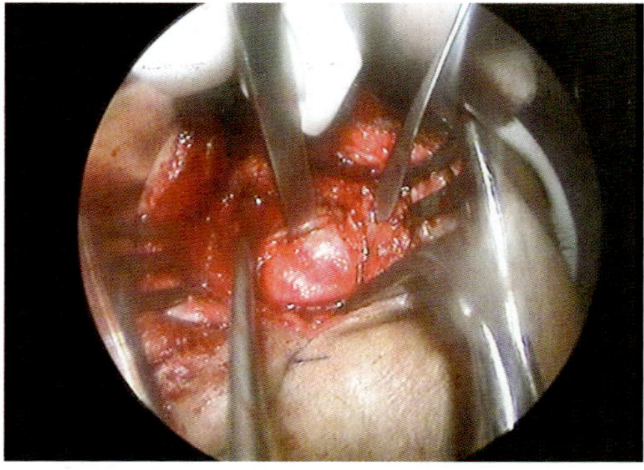

Fig. 62: Dissection of the ankylosed segment with the help of chisel hammer and drill

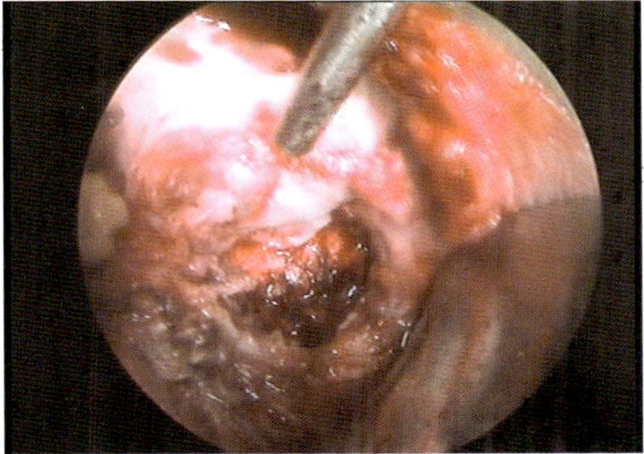

Fig. 63: Defect created after removal of ankylosed segment

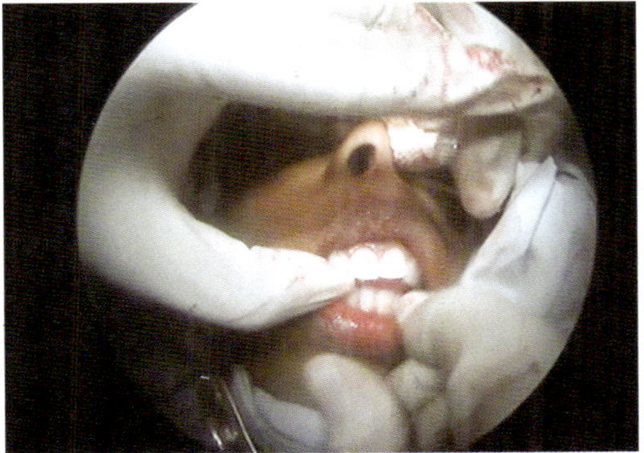

Fig. 64: Manipulation done to achieve the mouth opening

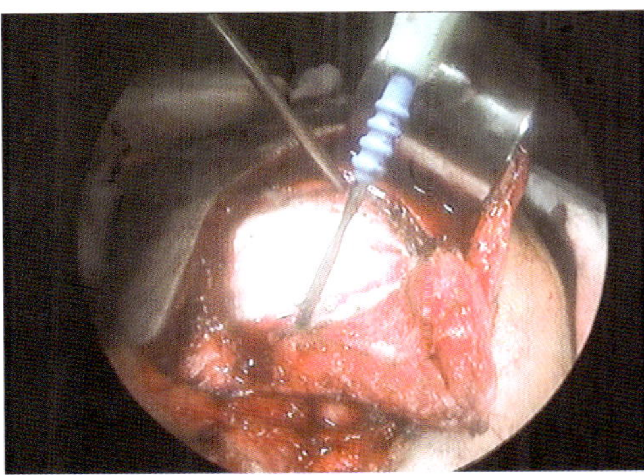

Fig. 65: Temporalis muscle myofacial flap elevated

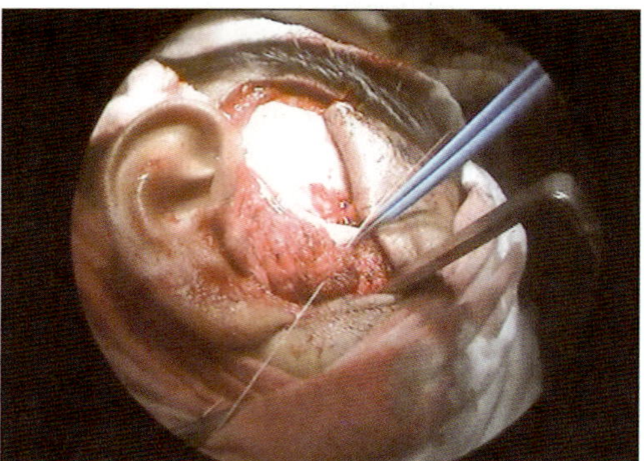

Fig. 66: Defected filled with the graft and secured with sutures

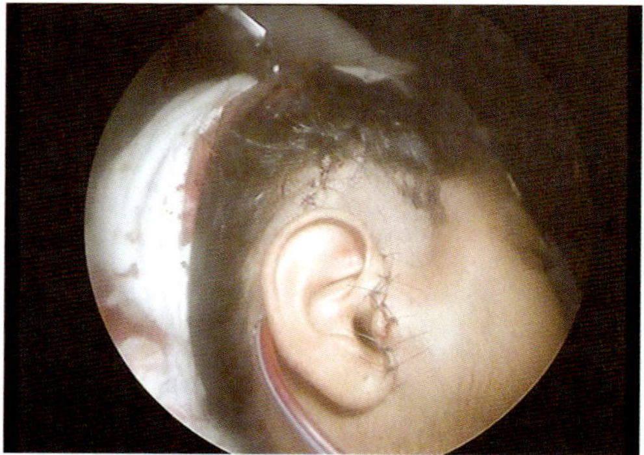

Fig. 67: Closure of wound in layers

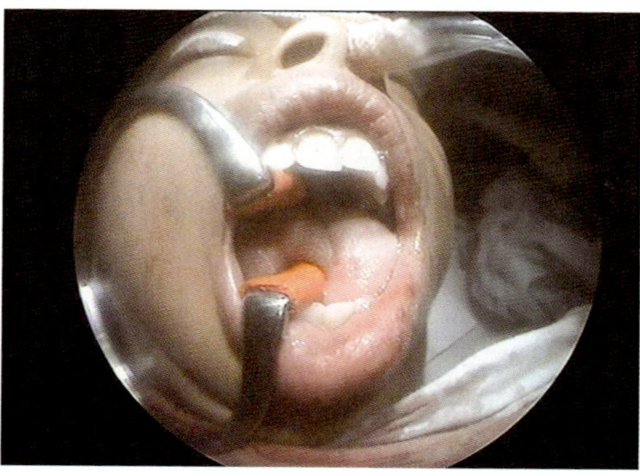

Fig. 68: Immediate postoperative picture showing 3.0 cm of mouth opening

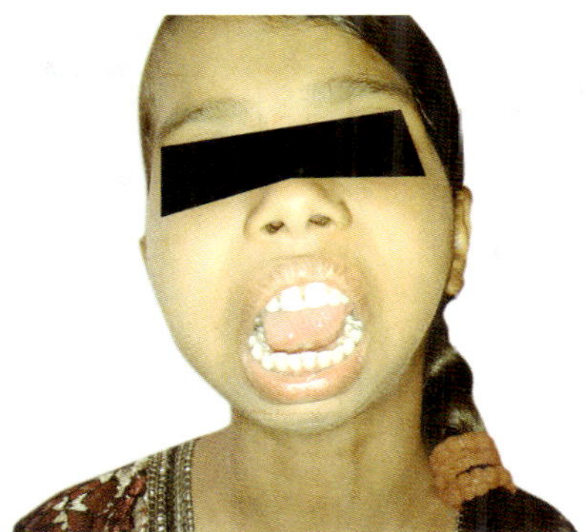

Fig. 69: Postoperative picture after 1 month showing adequate mouth opening (patient on active physiotherapy)

CASE 11: RECONSTRUCTION PLATE (COMMINUTED FRACTURE BODY MANDIBLE)

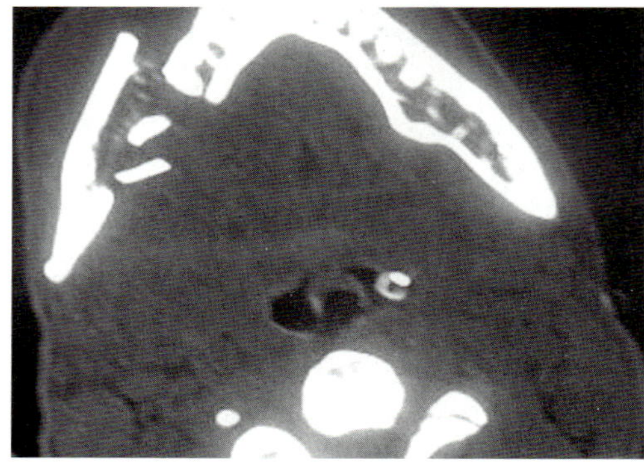

Fig. 70: CT scan showing comminuted fracture of body mandible involving both the buccal and lingual cortices on the right side

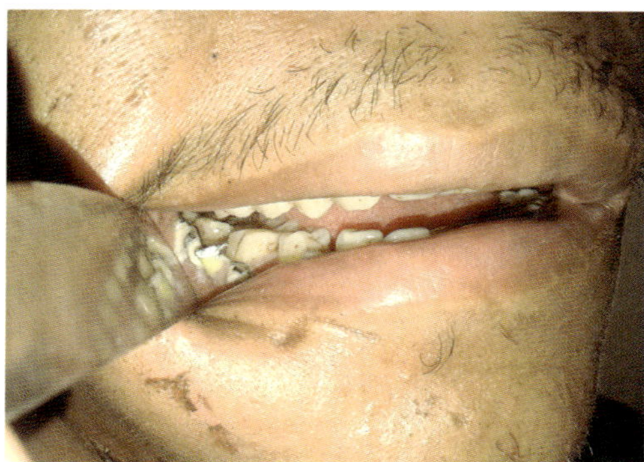

Fig. 71: Preoperative picture of the patient showing malocclusion (posterior open bite)

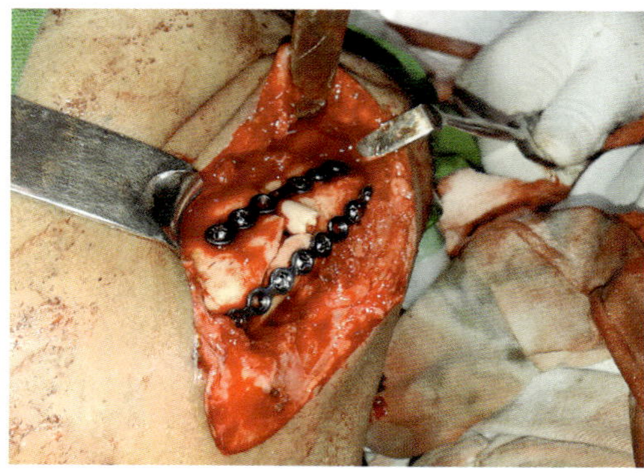

Fig. 72: Use of reconstruction plate at the lower border and mini-plate at upper border

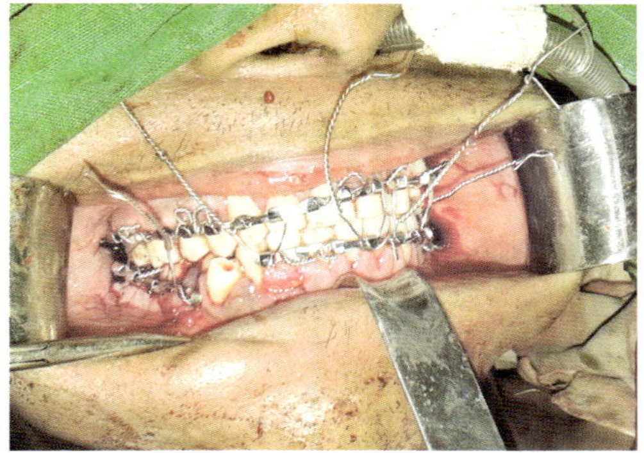

Fig. 73: Normal occlusion achieved with ORIF

CASE 12: RIB GRAFT

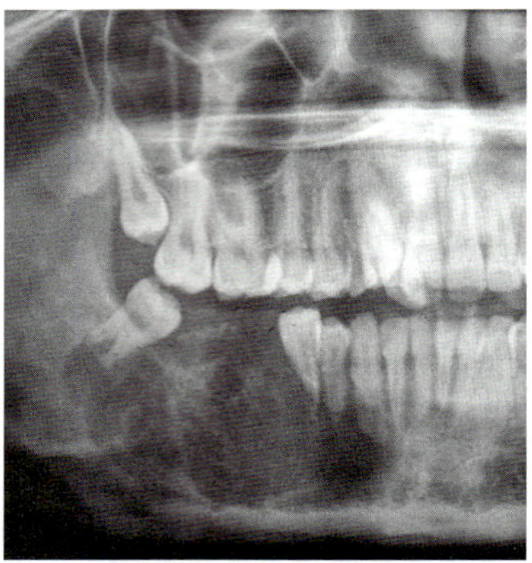

Fig. 74: OPG showing expansile bone cyst involving body and angle of the mandible on the right side

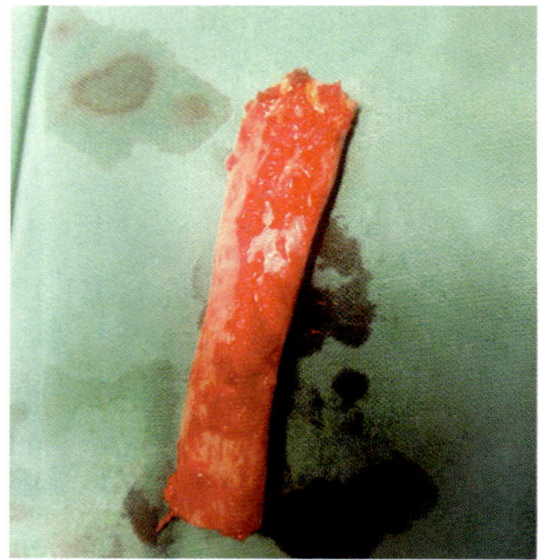

Fig. 75: Harvested rib graft

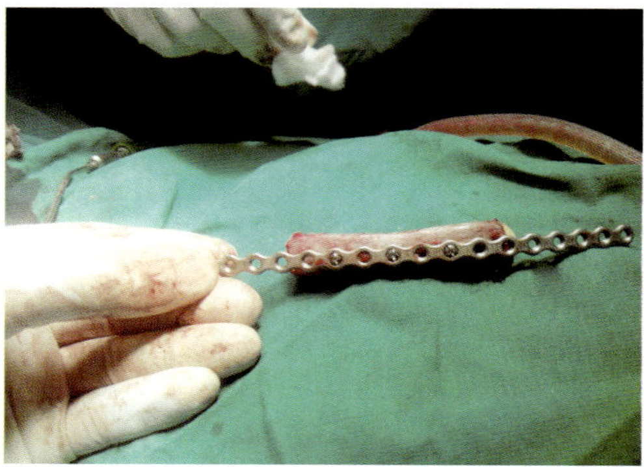

Fig. 76: Rib graft secured with reconstruction plate

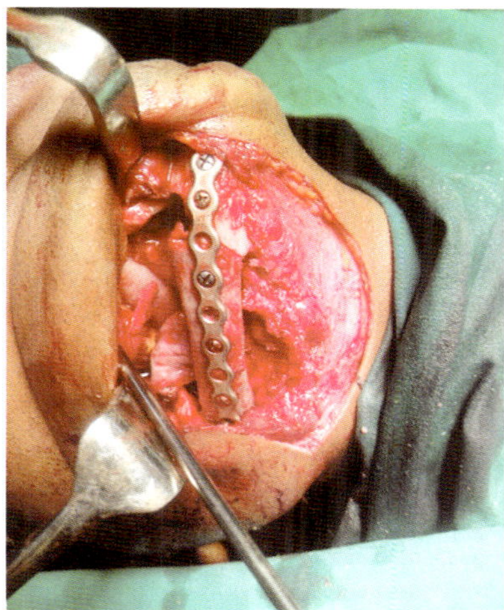

Fig. 77: Graft with reconstruction plate secured with adjacent mandible with minimal 2 screws on the adjacent bone

CASE 13: SYMPHYSIS FRACTURE (USE OF EXISTING WOUND)

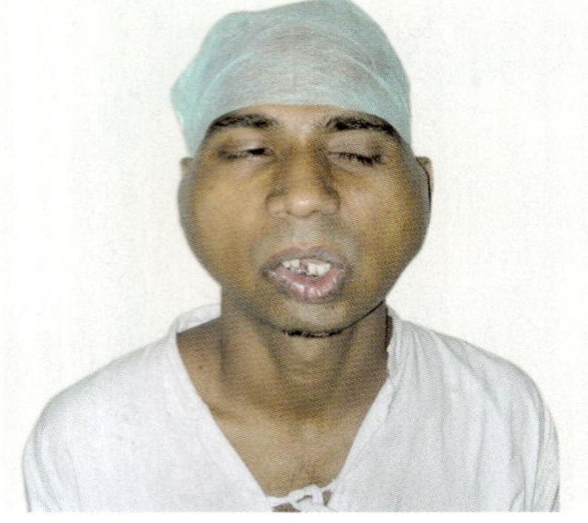

Fig. 78: Preoperative picture of a patient having symphysis fracture (posterior open bite and lacerated wound at submental region)

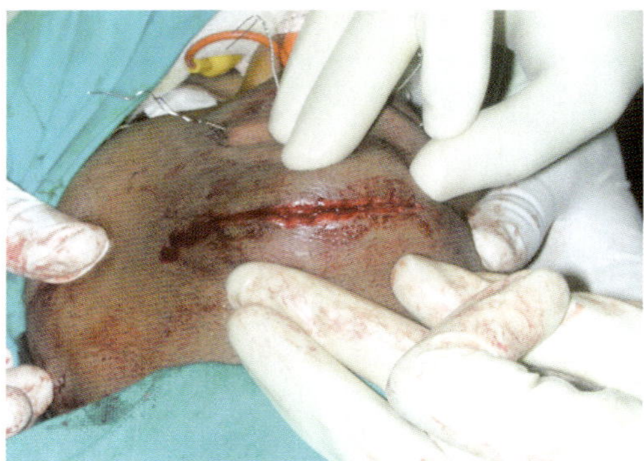

Fig. 79: Extrapolation of existing wound for the exposure of fracture site

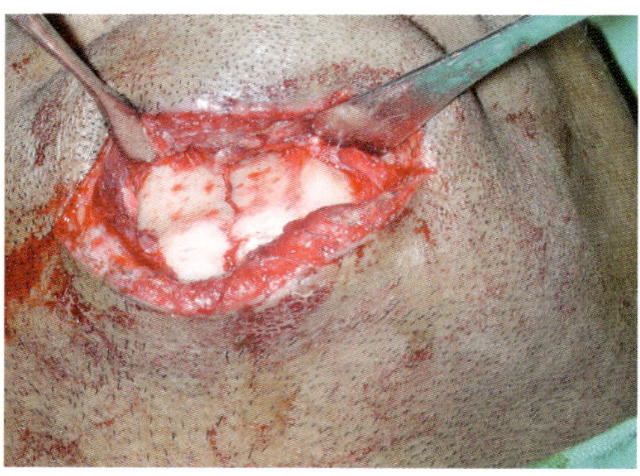

Fig. 80: Well-exposed fracture site

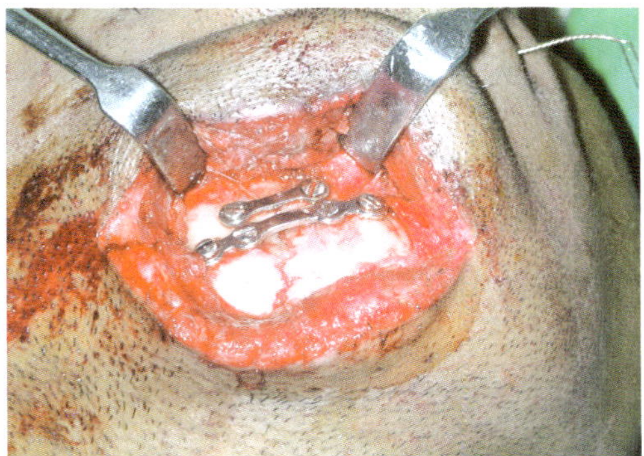

Fig. 81: Open reduction and internal fixature (ORIF) using mini-hole plates

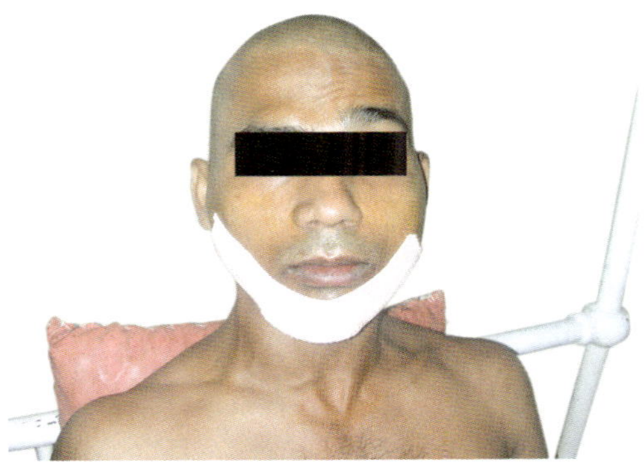

Fig. 82: Crepe bandange over the surgical site to avoid hematoma formation

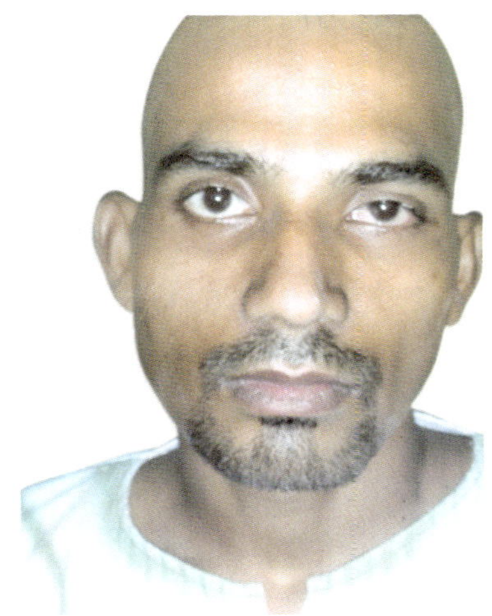

Fig. 83: Postoperative picture showing inconspicucus scar with normal facial symmetry

CASE 14: PARASYMPHYSIS FRACTURE (EXTRAORAL APPROACH)

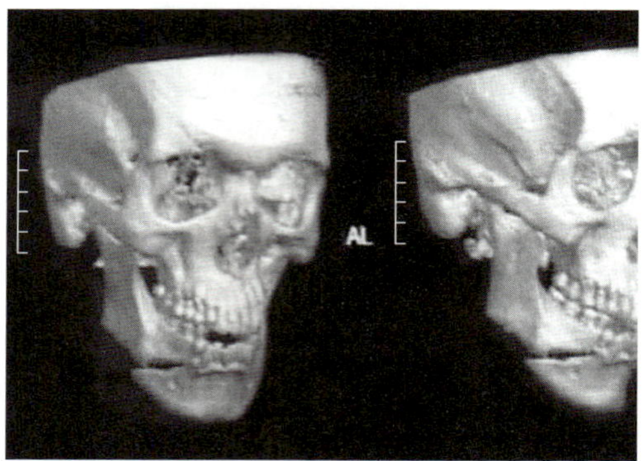

Fig. 84: Three-dimensional CT scan showing an oblique fracture line passing through parasymphysis region on the right side

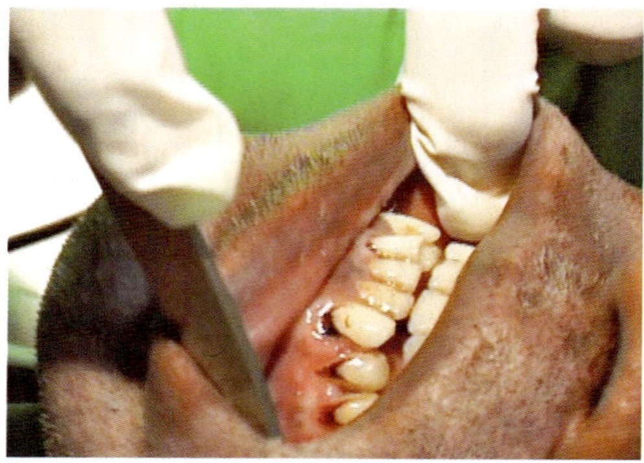

Fig. 85: Preoperative picture of the patient showing malocclusion

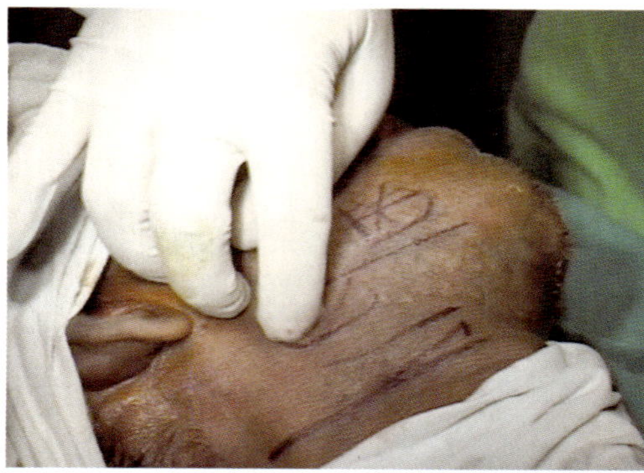

Fig. 86: Marking for submandibular incision (extraoral approach)

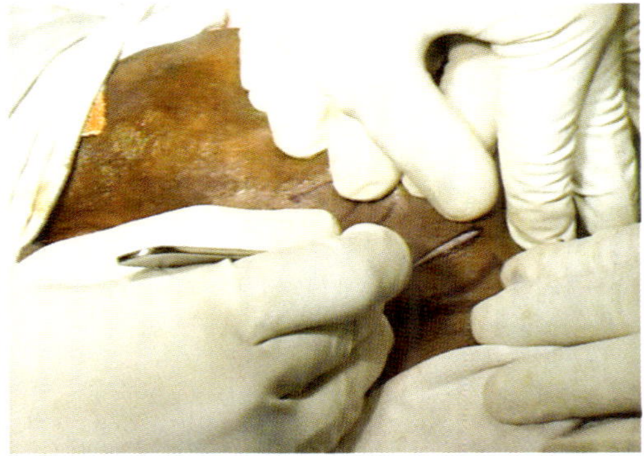

Fig. 87: Submandibular incision

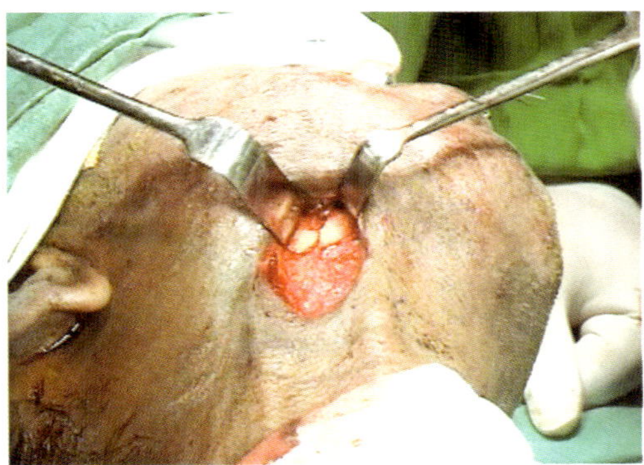

Fig. 88: Fracture site exposed after adequate dissection taking care not to injure the marginal mandibular nerve

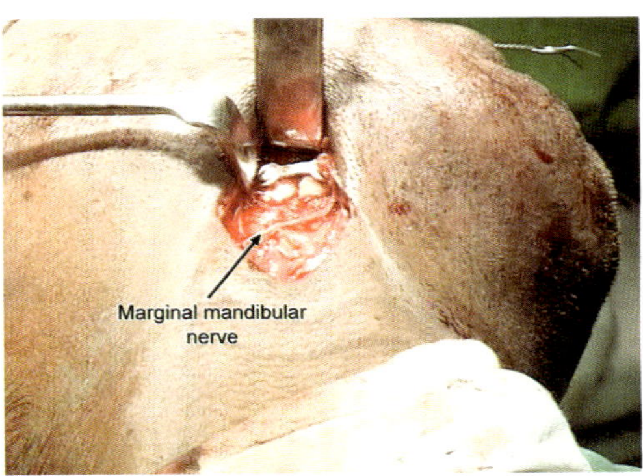

Fig. 89: Internal fixation done with mini-hole plates (marginal mandibular nerve well secured)

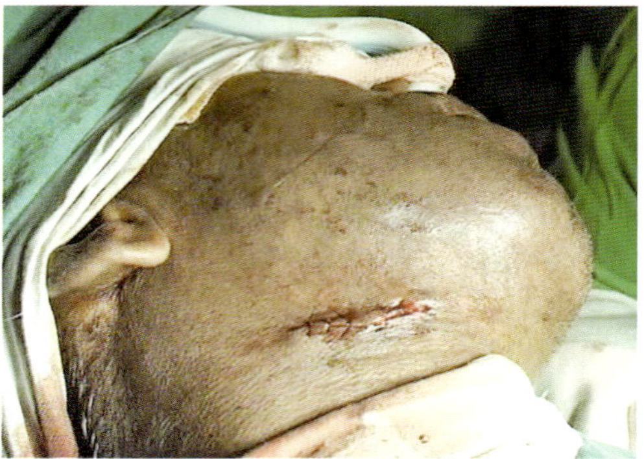

Fig. 90: Closure of wound in layers

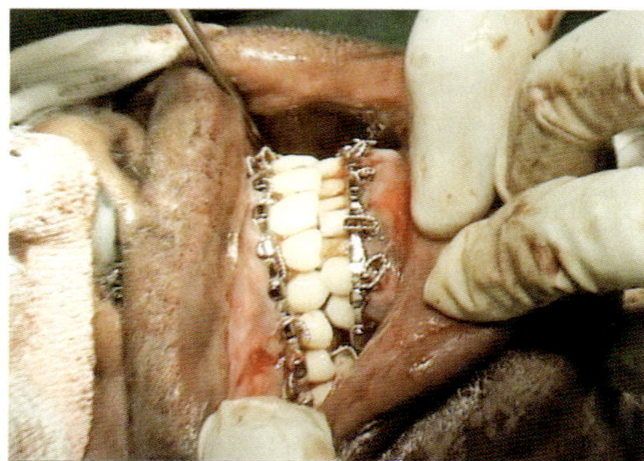

Fig. 91: Immediate postoperative normal occlusion

Index

Page numbers followed by '*f*' indicate figures.

F

G

N

O

S

T